Surviving Cancer

"This book contains a great deal of practical information that can be extremely helpful—and reassuring—to persons with cancer."

-Catherine S. Cordoba, M.S.W.
Director, Services & Rehabilitation
AMERICAN CANCER SOCIETY
California Division, Inc.

"This is an excellent comprehensive review of the cancer patient's emotions and environmental needs and the resources available for meeting them.
  Your section on 'Gathering and Maintaining Emotional Strength' is particularly inspiring and applicable to any interested individual concerned to live life more fully."

-Kathryn K. Himmelsbach, A.C.S.W.
Director, Service & Rehabilitation
AMERICAN CANCER SOCIETY
District of Columbia Division, Inc.

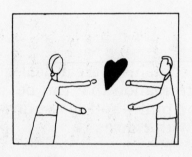

Illustrations by
Susan Davis

A Practical Guide
for Those Fighting
TO WIN!

Surviving
Cancer

Danette G. Kauffman

Foreword by Frederick G. Barr, M.D.

ACROPOLIS BOOKS LTD.
WASHINGTON, D.C.

ACROPOLIS BOOKS, LTD.
Colortone Building, 2400 17th St., N.W., Washington, D.C. 20009

Printed in the United States of America by
COLORTONE PRESS, Creative Graphics, Inc., Washington, D.C. 20009

Attention: Schools and Associations
ACROPOLIS books are available at quantity discounts with bulk purchase for educational, business, or sales promotional use. For information, please write to: SPECIAL SALES DEPARTMENT, ACROPOLIS BOOKS LTD., 2400 17th ST., N.W., WASHINGTON, D.C. 20009

**Are there Acropolis Books you want
but cannot find in your local stores?**
You can get any Acropolis book title in print. Simply send title and retail price, plus $2.00 for the first copy and $1.00 for each additional copy to cover mailing and handling costs. District of Columbia residents add applicable sales tax. Enclose check or money order only, no cash please, to:
ACROPOLIS BOOKS LTD., 2400 17th St., N.W., WASHINGTON, D.C. 20009.

The author gratefully acknowledges the permission to reprint from the following:

From the poem "Under Which Lyre" in *Shorter Poems*, by W. H. Auden. Reprinted by permission of Random House, Inc.

The excerpt on page 115 reprinted from *The Search for Signs of Intelligent Life in the Universe* by Jane Wagner. Copyright © 1986 by Jane Wagner, Inc. Reprinted by permission of Harper & Row, Publishers, Inc.

Library of Congress Cataloging-in-Publication Data
Kauffman, Danette G.,
  Surviving cancer.

  Includes index.
  1. Cancer—Patients—Rehabilitation.   2. Cancer—
Patients—Services for.   I. Title.   [DNLM: 1. Life Change
Events—popular works.   2. Medical Oncology—popular
works.   QZ 201 K21s]
RC261.K236   1987   616.99′4   87-1764
ISBN 0-87491-862-6 (pbk.)

This book was written for
Beverly
and for all those who, facing cancer,
keep fighting.

CONTENTS

Special thanks to those individuals who reviewed this manuscript and helped to make the information more complete, exact, and useful. They include: Frederick G. Barr, M.D., Medical Oncologist, Washington, D.C.; Catherine S. Cordoba, M.S.W., Director of Service and Rehabilitation, American Cancer Society, California Division; Kathryn K. Himmelsbach, A.C.S.W., Director, Service and Rehabilitation, American Cancer Society, D.C. Division; Barton L. Kraff, M.D., Metropolitan Psychiatric Group, Washington, D.C.; Basia Kulawiec, Program Director, The World Affairs Council of Maine; Jane Lewis, Health Communication Consultant; Margaret J. Lloyd, R.N., N.P., ON-C, Division of Hematology-Oncology, George Washington University Medical Center; and Nancy S. Mihocik, Teacher/Chemical Counselor, Rocky River High School, Rocky River, Ohio.

Thanks, also, to persons representing the many organizations, facilities, and other resources included in this book who willingly explained their services and clarified the information.

Leon A. LeBuffe, Ph.D., Executive Director, American Cancer Society, Los Angeles, and Diane Adams offered tremendous support as well as valuable critical perspective throughout this project. They encouraged me, reviewed every draft of the manuscript, and offered important insight, suggestions, and help.

Thanks to my parents, Gretchen and Dan Gentile, Deborah J. Childs, Paul Clifford, Jane D'Alelio, Susan Davis, Rebecca S. Wrenn, Edward L. Hunter, Geri Thoma, Sandra E. Vadney, Boyd Wanzer, and so many other friends and associates who, each in their own way, contributed personal and professional expertise, enthusiasm, and support to this project.

DGK

Modern medicine has become a highly technical field providing exciting new diagnostic tools and treatment modalities that have improved survival and quality of life. Along with this progress, however, goes a widening gap between patient and physician, a gap of language and understanding. The patient often leaves a physician's office facing a diagnostic test or a serious illness bewildered, not understanding or unable to obtain an explanation from the doctor.

As the public seeks to educate itself through awareness programs and publications that deal with medical issues at the lay level, these frustrations will be addressed. In addition, as acquiring second opinions becomes more readily acceptable within the medical profession, patients may feel reassured about a particular course of therapy and more a part of the decision-making process.

There have been many publications on cancer but few have provided the breadth of information encompassed in *Surviving Cancer*. Ms. Kauffman shares her experience and knowledge collected from the day a breast lump was discovered, through biopsy and surgery and later chemotherapy. There could be no better guide than one who has been there before and Ms. Kauffman, more appropriately than a physician, conveys the anxieties and side effects encountered in the treatment of cancer.

Surviving Cancer is a veritable treasure of information, names, addresses, and phone numbers for second opinions and resource material that encourage the patient to participate in his/her own care. Through my own reading of the manuscript, I found information that should be at the fingertips of all cancer specialists to provide for their patients.

As you read through this book you will find, as I have, that Danette Kauffman is a very special person whose love of life is translated into a fighting spirit that has allowed her to control a very dangerous disease. A particular suggestion may not apply to everyone, but her determination and will to live can only inspire others to fight for life.

Frederick G. Barr, M.D.
Medical Oncologist
Washington, D.C.

One of the greeting cards I opened after my second surgery for cancer startled me by its bare-bones simplicity: "Just remember to keep fighting."

The message in that greeting card helped focus my attention on the job I had to do—my role had to be an active one. I had to be working just as hard as the health professionals and caring just as much as my family and friends.

The tips, resources, and reminders in this book come out of one person's real life experiences fighting cancer and living with the uncertainty of cancer recurrence.

The book is organized for quick and easy reading and reference to a particular topic, chapter, or group of resources. The reader who reads from start to finish may notice several resources that appear in more than one chapter. This is intended to aid those readers who use this book to refer just to particular topics, chapters, or resource lists that are of special interest to them.

The resources in this book, no matter how useful, are not intended to be used as a substitute for competent medical care. Information about resources was verified by telephone or in writing right up to press time, but sometimes telephone numbers or other information may change without notice.

I hope you will find this book provides valuable resources that can make the job of fighting cancer—and winning—an enriching experience. I hope for you, too, the opportunity for growth that can come as a direct result of the struggle with serious illness.

DGK

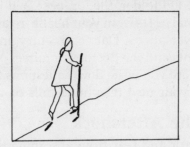

CHAPTER ONE

Immediate Mobilization

The news that it's cancer is devastating—no matter where or when or how you hear the news. Many people learn the news in the recovery room while they're still groggy from the anesthesia; others are told over the phone. Even under the best circumstances—surrounded by caring loved ones and taking as much time as necessary in the doctor's office—it's a tremendous shock and burden.

Here are some practical things you can do immediately to help organize and mobilize yourself for winning the fight against cancer.

Listening Effectively

Because you are most likely shocked and confused, take notes of everything your doctor says. If you are too caught up emotionally in the cancer diagnosis to concentrate on his or her message, bring a family member or trusted friend with you to listen and take notes.

If you or your friends are not good note takers, take a portable tape recorder to your initial meetings with your doctor, so that you can replay his or her comments later when you can listen without being distracted by your emotions.

Begin a portfolio folder, file, or loose-leaf notebook to keep factual and personal notes from your health-related appointments or telephone conversations. Date each entry. Include your questions and comments and the doctors' or nurses' responses. Keep a separate page where you write down questions to ask the doctors or nurses during your next telephone calls or visits.

Bracing for the Aftershock

Be aware that terror and fear from absorbing the shock of your cancer diagnosis—or starting follow-up chemotherapy or radiation treatment—can create a number of temporary reactions such as disorientation, chills, loss of appetite, dizziness, depression.

I have a clear recollection of feeling disoriented and confused for three or four days after receiving my cancer diagnosis. I could not concentrate on words that were spoken and I felt disconnected from life that was going on around me. I felt as if I were standing off to the side watching life happen rather than actually participating in it.

It took months for me to realize that this short-term disorientation and confusion were rooted in my depression and despair over the diagnosis and were not physical reactions to the anesthesia or surgery.

Several weeks after the diagnosis and surgery, when I began chemotherapy treatments, I experienced other frightening reactions—chills, loss of appetite, and total listlessness. My oncologist assured me that these were not side effects of the chemotherapy drugs. These reactions, it seems, came from my fear and depression over starting chemotherapy that was scary and unknown.

As I became accustomed to the chemotherapy regimen and saw that my life could continue even while I was on chemotherapy, the chills, anorexia, and hopelessness gradually eased.

Talking about these kinds of feelings, experiences, and apprehensions with family, friends, doctors, or counselors can help you move through these traumatic times and provide the hope to begin to cope with the scary road of uncertainties ahead.

Appointing a "Reader"

Ask one or more responsible friends or family members to act as your "readers." During the initial months of your diagnosis and treatment, you may find yourself deluged with books, articles, casebooks, recommendations on the best doctors, hospitals or cancer clinics, and other advice about what to do. This information can be very useful at specific times in your healing process. Your readers can divide up reading responsibilities, screen information, summarize it, and share specific information at particularly appropriate times.

Your readers can serve in another vital way, too, by helping you to avoid some of the frustration that comes from totally contradictory information. Because there are many unknowns about cancer, highly trained experts can, and often do, completely contradict each other about preferred treatment methods. It can be tremendously frustrating to be trying to get well by selecting the most appropriate treatment, only to have to sift through well-informed, well-documented articles that are in total disagreement. Your readers can examine the various articles and options, summarize the contradictory points, and present the essential facts to you in an "executive summary" fashion. You can then discuss the contradictory information with your physician who can give you the rationale for your treatment plan.

Besides reducing the frustration that comes from contradictory information, your readers can help minimize—*not* eliminate—the cold statistics that writers use to fortify their stories. It's much too easy to pick up these statistics, remember some of them out of context, and then allow the statistics to become overwhelming and depressing. Your readers can scan useful articles and report valuable points.

Getting Additional Information

Cancer Information Service

The National Cancer Institute maintains the Cancer Information Service network serving the entire United States to provide up-to-date information about cancer. Trained staff members (professionals and trained volunteers) operate this toll-free telephone inquiry service to give accurate, easy to understand answers to individual callers' questions. Free publications are available and can be mailed to callers to assist in answering questions.

The Cancer Information Service is for use by the general public, patients, families of patients, and health professionals. Staff members answer questions about such things as the causes and prevention of cancer; risk factors; the stages of the disease; treatment, detection, and diagnostic techniques; rehabilitation services; and the relationship of diet to cancer. While staff members do not make diagnoses or recommend treatments, they do offer a variety of useful resources and the latest information presented in simple, non-technical language.

Staff members also can provide information about medical facilities, physician referral suggestions, and other cancer-related resources—including names of National Cancer Institute-designated cancer centers, community hospitals with programs approved by The American College of Surgeons, and Second Opinion Centers.

Use the Cancer Information Service toll-free line, 1-800-4-CANCER, to contact the office serving your locale. Calls are answered Monday through Friday, 9 A.M. to 10 P.M. (Eastern Standard Time) and Saturday from 10 A.M. to 6 P.M. (Eastern Standard Time), either by local staff or by a central office, after hours. See the resources section of this chapter for additional information.

Nonprofit, Voluntary Health Organizations

Investigate the information and services provided by private, nonprofit voluntary health organizations. Local offices of the American Cancer Society provide information and guidance services. The Leukemia Society of America, The United Ostomy Association, and Make Today Count provide a variety of information or support services. Check your local telephone book for these numbers or see the Resources Section at the end of this chapter.

Local chapters of the nonprofit agencies mentioned above provide a variety of services, some of which might include individual or group counseling services, support groups, financial aid for the needy, transportation to medical treatments, home test kits, convalescent kits, referral suggestions, information brochures, and volunteer visitors to the home or hospital. (The visitors are usually persons who have successfully gone through exactly what you are facing.)

Putting the Computer to Work for Treatment Information

PDQ

A computerized information service, called PDQ (for physician data query), is available to provide doctors—and, beginning in 1986, patients—access to up-to-date cancer treatment information. The PDQ provides the latest technical information from major cancer treatment centers around the country and the world. The PDQ includes information about the staging system used to identify forms of cancer, options that are appropriate for a particular cancer at any given stage, and the prognosis for long-term survival. PDQ also provides information about where state-of-the-art treatment is being administered and what physicians in the requestor's area are offering these latest treatment methods.

Doctors have had this computerized information available for some time through the National Library of Medicine, but now patients can request this information themselves through the Cancer Information Service network. Contact your Cancer Information Service to request the computerized PDQ. Call the 1-800-4-CANCER toll-free line to speak with a trained staff member or volunteer who can request the PDQ for you.

Patients with a computer and modem can access the database directly, if they prefer. PDQ is available as an on-line service through the National Library of Medicine and through two commercial vendors, Mead Data Central's new medical information system—MEDIS—and BRS Saunders' System—Colleague. In California, the American Cancer Society can also provide information through a PDQ computer search.

Patients need the following technical information to request a computerized physician data query:

☐ Diagnosis, including the type and stage of cancer

☐ Where the primary cancer is located

☐ Cell type

☐ Address and telephone number of the physician providing treatment

The information in a PDQ was written for physicians and the text contains numerous abbreviations for medical terminology and medications. Since the computerized information is directed specifically to cancer treatment specialists, patients are advised to inform their doctor that they have requested the computerized treatment data and that they are having the report mailed directly to the doctor. After the doctor reads it and explains it thoroughly, the patient can review the treatment options with the doctor.

Patients who want to use their personal computer system to communicate with the database and obtain the PDQ on their own can complete an application for computer access. There is no charge to apply for an access code, but there is a charge for computer connection time while the search is being conducted. Call the National Library of Medicine MEDLARS Management Section, 301-496-6193, for an access code application form.

Bone Marrow Registry

A national program has recently begun to coordinate a computerized registry to search for matches between unrelated donors for bone marrow transplants. These centralized files will be available for use by approved transplant centers.

Bone marrow donor information currently exists in decentralized storage systems in a number of blood banks and transplant centers around the world. This bone marrow registry program ultimately will result in a nationwide network that will simplify and speed the search for unrelated donors for transplant matches. Ask your primary care physician for more information.

Determining Whom to Tell

Develop a strategy regarding who should be told about the diagnosis and how much information should be shared with these individuals.

The doctor I consulted for a second opinion about surgery cautioned me to be careful about sharing news about my health with many people. He said that experience showed that persons with cancer often fall victim to discrimination from employers and even from friends who find it very difficult to deal with news of a cancer diagnosis.

I was startled by his frankness and willingness to volunteer this information, and I found his ideas were worth thinking through. Together, my best friend and I decided on the few close friends we would tell; my friend handled the job of notifying them and asking them to keep the information private. I notified my parents and asked them not to share the information except with their closest friends who could give them much needed support.

At work, I told my management that I had a serious illness that was treatable but would require surgery and possible follow-up therapy. I assured them that all project deadlines would be met and that my staff and I would make sure the work continued on schedule. In addition to saying this to my own group executive, I gave the company's top human resources executive the same information and asked him to be sure that there was no effort to remove me from my position in my absence.

The information I shared at work was based on how I saw the corporate environment and what I wanted to accomplish with my department over the coming months. Others will find that their particular situation requires a different response. Options include everything from total openness about the illness with all friends and family to limited sharing or total silence. While telling friends and family may be difficult or cause discomfort, especially at first—for the patient or friends—the patient can realistically look ahead to the comfort and support these individuals can provide during what is often a lengthy illness.

Being Alert to Job Discrimination

If you feel you have been discriminated against because of your illness, you can contact community agencies that can help assist you in understanding your rights. The American Cancer Society is working on this problem of job discrimination. For example, in 1986 they funded an ongoing study of employment discrimination.

Also, they have produced a booklet entitled "Cancer: Your Job, Insurance, and the Law" that can offer general information and suggestions for action.

Deciding to Get Well

Richard Bloch, co-founder and Honorary Chairman of the Board of H&R Block, Inc., fought and beat inoperable lung cancer. He and his wife were determined to "lick this thing together" despite the fact that Bloch's surgeon gave him little or no hope of recovery and encouraged him to "get his estate in order."

In a personal interview for this book, Richard Bloch shared his experience facing cancer by reminding every cancer patient that "there is no type of cancer for which there is no treatment; and there is no type of cancer from which some people have not been cured." He encourages patients to "face the fact that we are all mortal and that we all die, but we're not statistics—we're persons. We can be involved and do everything possible to beat the disease."

Bloch advises newly-diagnosed cancer patients that "the largest, single killer of cancer patients is the belief that cancer is fatal." He advises patients to "get the finest medical treatment available and take that treatment all the way to its conclusion with no short cuts." He likewise encourages patients to decide as he and his wife did that "I can beat it; I have to get well."

Make the decision that you are going to get well. Look ahead to a very appealing future and picture yourself in it. Don't dwell on the scary unknown, but look beyond the surgery, chemotherapy, or radiation to days when you will be healthy again.

If you find making this decision hard or impossible, seek help from friends, family, a support group, or mental health professionals such as a psychologist, psychiatrist, social worker, or other counselor.

Taking Short Views

W. H. Auden, a twentieth century British poet, summed up his philosophy of coping with life in a playful, but concise phrase, "Read *The New Yorker*, trust in God; And take short views." The emphasis on keeping your mind focused on the immediate life around you is a healthy one for most persons, but especially for the person fighting cancer. Because there is really no way of knowing for sure just what the future holds, it seems wise to concentrate on living one day at a time with the best quality of life you can pack into that day. Take each lab test, pathology report, and chemotherapy or radiation treatment as it comes.

The most valuable experience I gained from the demanding effort of fighting cancer is to realize that each day and each hour and each moment is a precious treasure to be appreciated for its own uniqueness. This appreciation helps center you in the present moment, prepared to enjoy the experiences of the day.

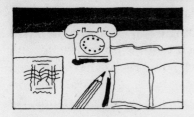

Resources for Immediate Mobilization

Be aware that the social service department of your local hospital may be able to provide you and your family with a variety of resources. These professionals can offer information about community, regional, and national resources; counseling services; problem-solving help; and related experience.

National Services and Information

National Cancer Institute
Cancer Information Service (CIS)
Building 31, Room 10A18
Bethesda, Maryland, 20892

The Cancer Information Service maintains a national telephone inquiry information network to provide medical and technical information, access to computerized state-of-the-art treatment information, assistance suggestions, and options about choices and treatment centers to callers from the general public, patients, families, and health professionals.

To order publications or to ask about specific cancer-related resources in your community, contact the Cancer Information Service information line—1-800-4-CANCER. The telephone information line is answered Monday to Friday, 9 A.M. to 10 P.M. (Eastern Standard Time) and Saturday from 10 A.M. to 6 P.M. (Eastern Standard Time), by extensively trained, certified volunteers and professional staff. Calls to local or regional Cancer Information Service offices are routed to the central office at the National Cancer Institute when local offices close for the day.

In Alaska, call 1-800-638-6070; in Oahu, Hawaii, call 524-1234 (call collect from neighboring islands). Spanish-speaking staff members are available during the day to callers from California, Florida, Georgia, Illinois, Northern New Jersey, New York City, and Texas.

American Cancer Society
90 Park Avenue
New York, New York 10016
212-736-3030

Fifty-eight Divisions and more than three thousand local units of the American Cancer Society offer a variety of services throughout the country including information and patient education, transportation, equipment loan or rental, dressings, and volunteer visitors programs.

The American Cancer Society provides its services at no charge to patients or family members. It receives no government support and relies on donations from the public.

Check your local telephone directory for the telephone number of your local unit of the American Cancer Society to ask about the programs and services they offer, including the following:

Information and Patient Education

Patients and their family members can receive information about cancer, community resources, and services available through the American Cancer Society as well as referrals to other resources.

I Can Cope is a group education program of the American Cancer Society for patients and their families to learn from health professionals about a variety of topics of interest to those facing cancer. The programs cover such areas as treatment methods, side effects of therapy, the role of nutrition for the cancer patient, and ways for patients and family members to cope with cancer. I Can Cope usually is offered in conjunction with hospital cancer centers.

Transportation Services

Volunteer drivers provide travel help for patients going to doctors' offices or hospitals for diagnosis, treatment, or rehabilitation. Some local units call this service the "Road to Recovery" program.

Home Care Items

Patients can receive useful items at home to simplify their experience fighting and recovering from cancer. Durable medical equipment can be provided based on the physician's recommendation and the patient's need and other circumstances.

Volunteer Visitor Programs

Trained visitors offer practical information and emotional support, but not medical information. Usually the visitors are recovered patients who have successfully faced similar experiences with cancer.

. **Reach to Recovery**—a short-term program that puts women newly diagnosed with breast cancer in contact with women who have coped well with their own breast cancer experience and who have been trained by the American Cancer Society. The trained volunteers demonstrate by their presence their successful recovery and provide emotional support and practical information on rehabilitation. New patients can share their feelings and concerns about the treatment and recovery stages, about using temporary or permanent prostheses, and about reconstruction options. Literature for family members of breast cancer patients is also available.

Ostomy Patient Rehabilitation Program—services vary. Contact your local American Cancer Society office or division for information about local resources and services. The United Ostomy Association cooperates with the American Cancer Society in providing a visitors' program and educational materials.

Laryngectomy Patient Rehabilitation Program—this program offers helpful information and support to the laryngectomy patient before and after surgery. Some local clubs, which may call themselves The Lost Chord, offer speech lessons. The International Associaton of Laryngectomies cooperates with the American Cancer Society to provide trained volunteers.

CanSurmount or Can Support—a patient-to-patient, one-on-one visitor program of the American Cancer Society for cancer patients and their families to meet and talk with trained volunteers who provide emotional support and useful information.

Guestroom Program

Patients and family members who need to travel to treatment facilities and who lack financial resources for the overnight stay can be assisted. Westin Hotels and Resorts in the United States and other hotels and motels are cooperating with the American Cancer Society to make hotel accommodations available at no cost to patients and their families for those patients who have to travel outside their home area for treatment. Accommodations are subject to a hotel's projection of vacancy. Normally, the offer is limited to six consecutive weeks. Parking and room occupancy tax may or may not be complimentary based on local circumstances.

Arrangements can only be made by contacting your local American Cancer Society office, not Westin Hotels and Resorts. Your local American Cancer Society office will handle all arrangements for your accommodations and provide any further instructions.

Childhood Cancer Program

This American Cancer Society program is designed to provide information to parents, siblings, teachers, and classmates about the special needs of children with cancer. Information is also available to health professionals about the advances made in treating pediatric cancers.

Some areas have summer camps sponsored by the American Cancer Society to provide recreation and contact within a medical support environment for children with cancer. Some areas also provide this support and recreational environment for siblings and parents.

Candlelighters Childhood Cancer Foundation
2025 I Street, N.W., Suite 1011
Washington, D.C. 20006
202-659-5136

Candlelighters is an international network of more than two hundred groups throughout the world that provides support and educational information for parents of children with cancer. The organization also provides a long-term survivors network. This private, nonprofit foundation produces a quarterly newsletter, youth newsletter, annotated bibliography and resource guide, and regular progress reports with information about treatment advances. The national office receives support from the American Cancer Society.

The Leukemia Society of America
733 Third Avenue
New York, New York 10017
212-573-8484
Contact: Public Information and Education

Fifty-seven chapters across the United States provide literature and audiovisual programs about the disease and its treatment. This nonprofit agency offers modest financial assistance, up to a maximum of $750 per year, to assist outpatients with medical payments and transportation costs. Some chapters offer support groups for patients and families. The Society publishes a quarterly newsletter and "Update" reports on its research program and treatment advances.

Make Today Count
P.O. Box 222
Osage Beach, Missouri 65065
314-348-1619

Make Today Count has more than two hundred local chapters in the United States, Canada, Germany, and Australia to provide emotional support to patients with life-threatening illnesses and their families. Though local chapters vary, they offer such services as group meetings, a telephone "buddy" system, home and hospital visits, educational workshops, emergency transportation or baby sitting services, and printed materials. This nonprofit organization is dedicated to helping all persons improve the quality of their life, identify emotional needs in order to learn to deal with them, and respond to serious illness openly and honestly.

Contact the national office for the local chapter in your area or to be matched to a buddy who can offer understanding and support by telephone or mail.

International Ronald McDonald Houses
Golin/Harris Communications, Inc.
500 North Michigan Avenue
Chicago, Illinois 60611
312-836-7114

Ronald McDonald Houses are operated in more than one hundred cities in the United States, Canada, Australia, and Europe to provide housing for parents and families of seriously ill children who are hospitalized. Contact the national number to obtain the address and telephone number of the Ronald McDonald House in your area or ask the social service department of your hospital about this or other housing options. Houses have different policies and operating guidelines. A fee of $5 to $15 per night per family is requested, but if the family cannot pay, the fee can be waived.

The United Cancer Council, Inc.
650 East Carmel Drive, Suite 340
Carmel, Indiana 46032
317-844-6627

The United Cancer Council has thirty-six local affiliate offices in twelve states, many operating under names different from United Cancer Council. Contact the national office for the local affiliate in your area or for information or referral services.

Local affiliates vary, but they usually offer printed materials about the disease and its treatment, information about community services, programs, and support groups for patients and their families, loan of equipment such as walkers, hospital beds, or wheelchairs to aid in caring for cancer patients at home, and transportation to doctors' offices and treatment centers. In addition, some agencies offer programs to quit smoking or the use of smokeless tobacco products, cancer detection clinics, breast self-examination clinics, professional counseling services, and direct financial assistance to help pay for prescriptions and treatments.

The United Cancer Council publishes *The Coordinator*, a bimonthly newsletter distributed through the local agencies.

United Ostomy Association
2001 West Beverly Boulevard
Los Angeles, California 90057
213-413-5510

More than six hundred and fifty chapters throughout the United States and Canada provide a variety of services. These include such services as information and printed materials, visitors to hospitals to support new patients, financial assistance, support groups, and transportation to doctors' offices and hospitals.

The national office publishes *Ostomy Quarterly* for members. This private, nonprofit organization supports efforts for improved equipment, supplies, and management techniques. Contact the national headquaters office for the telephone number of the local chapter in your area.

National Board of the Y.W.C.A.
ENCORE
726 Broadway
New York, New York 10003
212-614-2844

ENCORE is an exercise and discussion program for women who have had breast cancer surgery. The exercise consists of floor work and water exercises when a pool is available. Group discussions focus on the common concerns related to breast cancer, mastectomy, and other surgery for breast cancer. Contact the national office or your local Y.W.C.A.

Breast Cancer Advisory Center
P.O. Box 224
Kensington, Maryland 20895

An organization concerned with all aspects of breast cancer— detection, diagnosis, treatment, rehabilitation, and continuing care. Request free information by mail.

National Association of Meal Programs
204 E Street, N.W.
Washington, D.C. 20002
202-547-6157
Contact: Michael Giuffrida, Administrative Director

Communities have different names for the service of delivering meals to the sick, disabled, frail, elderly, or others who are homebound. Most common names are Meals on Wheels, M.O.W., and Mobile Meals. Contact the national association for information.

Visiting Nurse Associations

More than five hundred Visiting Nurse Associations exist throughout the country to provide a variety of home health care services. Check your local telephone directory for information about an organization in your locale. Also see Chapter Ten, Working Toward Quality Living, for more information.

National Women's Health Network
224 7th Street, S.E.
Washington, D.C. 20003
202-543-9222

The National Women's Health Network is a public interest organization that can provide current information on a variety of women's health matters. Information packets on cervical and breast cancer are available. Make request by mail.

Computerized Cancer Treatment Data Base Inquiry

Patients can request directly a PDQ (physician data query) or computerized printout of information about state-of-the-art cancer treatment methods for their particular kind and stage of cancer. Make requests for the data base search through your local Cancer Information Service office. Call 1-800-4-CANCER.

Patients need to be able to give specific information about the diagnosis, including the type and stage of cancer, where the primary cancer is located, and the cell type. Because the information in the PDQ is technical, patients are strongly advised to have their doctor request the PDQ or have the computerized printout of treatment data mailed directly to the doctor's office.

Patients with their own communicating computer terminal can obtain the PDQ by dialing in directly to the data base. Contact the National Library of Medicine MEDLARS Management Section for an access code application form, 301-496-6193. There is no charge to apply, but computer connection time is billed at an hourly rate. PDQ is available as an on-line service through the National Library of Medicine and through two commercial vendors, Mead Data Central's new medical information system—MEDIS—and BRS Saunders' System—Colleague. In California, the American Cancer Society can also provide information through a PDQ computer search.

Long Distance Transportation Services

The Corporate Angel Network (CAN)
Building One
Westchester County Airport
White Plains, New York 10604
914-328-1313
Hours: 8:30 A.M. to 4:30 P.M., Monday-Friday

The Corporate Angel Network is a nonprofit agency that matches unused seats on corporate aircraft with cancer patients needing transportation to medical care. Transportation is provided within the United States and only to or from a recognized cancer center or hospital for diagnosis, second opinion, or treatment. Treatment must be of the type approved by the American Cancer Society or the National Cancer Institute.

A patient needs authorization from the doctor (by letter or telephone call), must be able to walk up the aircraft stairs, and must use no life support systems. Patients need to provide the Corporate Angel Network with their doctor's name and telephone number and their telephone number and destination. Patients may be accompanied by another person if a second seat is available.

Patients are encouraged to contact the Corporate Angel Network seven to ten days in advance of travel and to book commercial transportation as a back-up.

Regional Services and Information

In addition to the resources that follow, check with the Cancer Information Service, your local American Cancer Society office, and the social service department of your hospital for detailed information about regional and community resources.

Cancer Care, Inc.
National Cancer Care Foundation, Inc.
1180 Avenue of the Americas
New York, New York 10036
212-302-2400
Contact: Social Services

This private, nonprofit agency serves patients and their families in the metropolitan New York area, including New York City, southern Connecticut, and all of New Jersey.

Cancer Care, Inc., offers a wide range of individual and group counseling for patients and their families. The agency assists with long-term planning and cost-sharing to help meet patients' needs for home care and costs for transportation to chemotherapy or radiation treatments. Cancer Care, Inc., operates a Friendly Visitors Program that provides volunteers to visit, chat, and "be with" patients. In addition, the agency offers counseling and other assistance to businesses whose employees are dealing with their own cancer diagnosis or one within the family. Cancer Care, Inc., provides education and training programs for health professionals and help with second opinions and coping skills for patients and families.

NEED

Meets at various locations in the metropolitan Baltimore, Maryland, area

301-685-1460 or 301-358-0707

Contact: NEED Program

A structured, ten-week program of health education for women who have had mastectomies. The two-hour classes concentrate on Nutrition, Exercise, Education, and Discussion, with each portion of the program led by a trained health professional who follows a set curriculum.

A nutrition specialist presents information on such topics as dietary guidelines and how to develop an appropriate diet. A physical therapist leads a discussion and presents information on such topics as the physical effects of surgery, stress management, how persons may feel on chemotherapy. The physical therapist also offers a home exercise program. Discussions focus on emotional, physical, and social aspects of breast cancer; coping mechanisms; and communicating with doctors, children, and other family members.

Call for printed information and to register for spring or fall classes. Participants are asked to have had their surgery at least six weeks before attending classes.

Started by a grant from Johns Hopkins Oncology Center, this program is now sponsored by the Y.W.C.A. of Greater Baltimore, The National Council of Jewish Women, The American Cancer Society, and Reach to Recovery.

No charge.

Cancer Counseling Institute
7312 Millwood Road
Bethesda, Maryland 20817

301-986-9273

The Cancer Counseling Institute provides information and materials, workshops, and individual and group counseling for patients and families. The Institute also offers training programs for psychotherapists, nurses, and other health professionals. It serves patients and trainees in the metropolitan Washington area and those outside the area who elect to come to Washington the third weekend of each month.

Today Our Understanding of Cancer is Hope (TOUCH)
St. Vincent's Hospital
2701 Ninth Court South
Birmingham, AL 35201
205-939-7000
Contact: Louis Josof

Nine chapters in Alabama and the southeast region provide support groups, educational and wellness programs, and friendly visitors for patients, their families, and friends. Trained volunteers visit patients at home, hospitals, outpatient clinics, or physicians' offices. Support groups are led by counselors, social workers, oncology nurses, and/or pastoral care representatives.

The Wellness Community
1235 Fifth Street
Santa Monica, California 90401
213-393-1415

The Wellness Community offers a variety of psychological and social programs free of charge to cancer patients, their families, and friends. Support groups for patients, led by licensed psychotherapists, present methods for dealing with physical and emotional problems associated with fighting cancer in order for patients to regain control of their lives.

Other Wellness Community offerings include guided imagery/visualization sessions, laughter exchanges, nutrition and other educational discussions, and special workshops.

Books

Getting Well Again, O. Carl Simonton, Stephanie Matthews-Simonton, James L. Creighton, Bantam, 1978.

This controversial book encourages patients with cancer to participate actively in getting well again through a clearly defined program of exercise, relaxation, visual imagery, and psychotherapy in addition to traditional medical intervention. The authors hypothesize a link between stress and the onset of cancer and outline typical psychological factors they have observed which are common to individuals who have developed cancer.

The book is considered controversial because other researchers, including those of the American Cancer Society, do not see a link between stress, personality, and the onset of cancer. Aids such as exercise, relaxation, imagery, and psychotherapy that the Simontons and Creighton propose as supplements to a full medical program are *not* controversial. In fact, relaxation therapy and hypnosis are becoming widely accepted as helpful practices for cancer patients.

The positive, downright encouraging message of this book allows individuals with cancer to see the benefits that can come out of illness and to examine their priorities and set goals to achieve a high quality future.

Choices: Realistic Alternatives in Cancer Treatment, Marion Morra and Eve Potts, Avon, 1980; revised 1987.

A comprehensive reference book about cancer that includes detailed information about selecting a doctor and hospital, understanding what cancer is, and the various diagnostic tests and treatments, including surgery, radiation, chemotherapy, immunotherapy, and experimental and unproven treatments. A major portion of the book provides lists and resources of where to get medical help.

The American Cancer Society Cancer Book: Prevention, Detection, Diagnosis, Treatment, Rehabilitation, Cure, Arthur I. Holleb, M.D., editor, Doubleday, Garden City, New York, 1986.

The American Cancer Society Cancer Book is a comprehensive collection of 35 separate essays offered by distinguished persons in the particular area being presented. The 650-page book is written in a consistently clear, easy to read style. Each chapter presents a thorough discussion of a particular issue, such as "Living With Cancer," "Cancer Prevention: Steps You Can Take," "Modern Cancer Therapy," "Coping With Problems Related to Cancer and Cancer Treatment," "Experimental Treatments and Research," and "Questionable Cancer Remedies."

The essays are organized around two major themes: "Where We Stand in the Battle With Cancer," and "Specific

Cancers and Their Treatment." Most essays include a summary section and a few chapters provide a list of related reading materials for further information. Some chapters offer specific, practical advice such as "Coping With Cancer Treatment Problems," which lists suggestions for handling a variety of treatment-related difficulties.

A 12-page "Directory of Resources" appendix provides addresses for the 58 American Cancer Society Chartered Divisions, addresses and telephone numbers for Comprehensive Cancer Centers, and contact information and a description of organizations that offer support, education, rehabilitation, home health care, and other services. *The American Cancer Society Cancer Book* also includes a glossary of terms and a particularly useful index.

Fighting Cancer, Richard Bloch and Annette Bloch, Cancer Connection, Inc., 1985.

Fighting Cancer presents technical information about the disease, resources for finding available treatment information, and numerous other suggestions for successfully taking action to defeat the disease. The book includes a quiz to help patients assess their mental attitude for fighting their cancer and a section answering "Twenty-Five Most Asked Questions."

Cancer, There's Hope, Richard Bloch and Annette Bloch, Cancer Connection, Inc., 1981.

Cancer, There's Hope, tells the grueling, but successful and rewarding story of Richard Bloch's fight against lung cancer. The book provides lists of Comprehensive Cancer Centers and a useful glossary of terms related to cancer.

Booklets and Fact Sheets

The National Cancer Institute and the American Cancer Society provide numerous publications free of charge for the general public, patients, and families of patients. Separate, scholarly publications are also available for health professionals.

To request National Cancer Institute publications use the toll-free phone number, 1-800-4-CANCER. A few of the available publications are:

"What You Need to Know. . .," a series of booklets about different types of cancer. Request the booklet based on your particular need.

"Chemotherapy and You: A Guide to Self-Help During Treatment"

"Radiation Therapy: A Treatment for Early Stage Breast Cancer"

"Eating Hints: Recipes and Tips for Better Nutrition During Cancer Treatment"

"Answers to Your Questions About Metastatic Cancer"

"Diagnosing Cancer: A Glossary of Medical Terms"

"Taking Time: Support for People with Cancer and the People Who Care About Them"

"Control of Cancer Pain Fact Sheet"

"Radiation Therapy for Cancer Fact Sheet"

Contact your local American Cancer Society office to request publications such as:

"Answering Your Questions About Cancer"

"Nutrition for Patients Receiving Chemotherapy and Radiation Treatment"

"Questions and Answers about Pain Control"

"What Is Chemotherapy?"

"Listen With Your Heart: Talking With the Cancer Patient"

"Cancer Facts and Figures"

"Cancer: Your Job, Insurance, and the Law"

"If You Find a Lump in Your Breast"

"Talking With Your Doctor"

Videotapes

"Fight for Your Life: Survival Techniques for Those With Cancer," is a comprehensive, motivational program to teach survival techniques to those with cancer or other life-threatening illnesses. The two-hour tape contains information and exercises for relaxation, visualization, meditation, and personal affirmation. The tape is available for $65, plus $3 shipping, by calling 1-800-225-5669, or by writing Varied Directions, Inc., 63 Elm Street, Camden, Maine 04843.

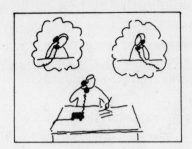

CHAPTER TWO

Getting a
Second Opinion
and Treatment

Elmo Zumwalt III, Vietnam naval officer and son of Admiral Elmo R. Zumwalt, Jr., fought a rare combination of two completely different cancers of the lymphatic system—Hodgkin's disease as well as non-Hodgkin's lymphoma. After a three-year battle consisting of treatment with chemotherapy, radiation therapy, and a grueling bone-marrow transplant, Zumwalt is hopeful that all signs point toward having beaten the diseases.

The younger Zumwalt reaches out for opportunities, such as through his book *My Father, My Son*, the interview aired on the ABC-TV program "20/20," and his personal interview for this book, to share his experiences and information so that other patients can profit from them. He is a staunch believer in getting a second opinion, a third opinion, or as many opinions as needed to reach a consensus on the best treatment program. He reminds patients to be open-minded and diligent in seeking additional opinions. Especially with rare forms of cancer such as his, he reminds patients that it may be necessary to get the diagnosis and treatment options reviewed and confirmed by a number of experts.

"Besides seeking a second or third opinion," Zumwalt adds, "achieve some consensus about the diagnosis and recommended treatment. In addition, find the best and most dedicated team of doctors and nurses.

"Find out where they are doing the premier work on your kind of cancer," Zumwalt advises. "Keep asking questions to find out which institutions are setting the standards for treatment that others are following.

"It's not necessary to think just in terms of finding the best doctors within your city or state," Zumwalt points out, "When you're thinking about your life, go find the very best medical team wherever they are!"

Elmo Zumwalt's belief in taking time and effort to find the best medical treatment—wherever it may be—is strongly seconded by Hamilton Jordan, White House Chief of Staff during the Carter administration.

When Jordan was diagnosed with lymphoma (the same type as Zumwalt's), he immediately gathered information about proposed treatment at several medical centers, as well as statistics about those medical centers' success rates. His decision about where to go for treatment became clearer when he learned that one medical center's 35 percent success rate with this particular kind of cancer, could be an 85 percent success rate at another medical center he was considering.

Now in remission for almost a year, Jordan reminds other patients to learn from such experiences and "manage your own medical care in order to find the best place to be treated for your disease."

Elmo Zumwalt's and Hamilton Jordan's belief in the value of getting other expert opinions is fully supported by the American Cancer Society, and most other nonprofit agencies, which encourage all patients to seek a second opinion about any treatment for cancer, whether it involves surgery, chemotherapy, radiation therapy, or other treatments.

Many insurance programs, in their effort to reduce the rising cost of health care, will pay 100 percent of the costs associated with getting a second opinion about any proposed surgery. Some insurance carriers feel so strongly about the need for a second opinion about certain surgical procedures—whether the condition is related to cancer or something else—that a second opinion on surgery is mandatory. Some insurance companies reduce the benefits they will pay when a patient does not seek a second opinion about surgery.

Gathering Materials for Review

You will need to request and gather for review all materials having to do with your diagnosis. These would include such things as your medical history, a full medical report from your physician, any available pathology reports, slides from biopsies, and x rays or scans. Some physicians and medical centers providing a second opinion may request a referral letter from your doctor as well.

Copies of lab tests or pathology slides usually are available for a nominal fee from the lab or hospital that performed the tests. Contact the lab or hospital during regular business hours. If you have difficulty getting the materials you need, ask for assistance from the office staff of the doctor who requested the tests.

Doctors or medical facilities offering a second opinion may request that some tests be performed again and that biopsy slides, x rays, or scans be re-examined to verify the accuracy of initial test findings.

Locating the Place to Get a Second Opinion or Treatment

Ask the Cancer Information Service of the National Cancer Institute, your local office of the American Cancer Society, National Cancer Institute-designated Cancer Centers, Second Opinion Centers, the American College of Surgeons, or your family doctor for advice on selecting a hospital, cancer center, or specialist to provide a second opinion or cancer treatment. These resources are described in detail below. Also see the resources section at the end of this chapter for specific addresses and telephone numbers.

In addition, you may want to speak with individuals who have gone through what you are facing to get their suggestions and recommendations. If so, contact one of the agencies listed in the resources section of Chapter One for other referral ideas.

Clinical Center of the National Institutes of Health

The Clinical Center of the National Institutes of Health provides treatment to patients whose diagnosis meets specific requirements of a particular research study or protocol. Patients must be referred by their physician. See the resources section at the end of this chapter for more information about the Clinical Center.

National Cancer Institute-designated Cancer Centers

The National Cancer Institute provides government grants to treatment centers that pass an ongoing peer review panel examining the overall quality of the cancer center's accomplishments. This peer review system means that cancer centers listed as "National Cancer Institute-designated Cancer Centers" demonstrate high quality work in areas such as cancer research, prevention, detection, diagnosis, treatment, and professional and volunteer training and education.

See the list of National Cancer Institute-designated Cancer Centers in the resources section at the end of this chapter or contact the Cancer Information Service at 1-800-4-CANCER.

Second Opinion Centers

Second Opinion Centers exist across the country to provide patients with access to a team of various specialists—including pathologists, surgeons, oncologists, radiologists, and others—who can examine the patient's medical history and other facts to provide a sound second opinion about the best course of treatment.

The hospitals and clinics listed as Second Opinion Centers have agreed to participate within a general framework pioneered by the R. A. Bloch Cancer Management Center to invite patients and their family members to be present and ask questions as the interdisciplinary team analyzes and discusses the case. While review boards of this kind are fairly common for doctors and other health professionals to be a part of, it is not common for patients or their families to be able to participate in or attend these meetings.

If you want to be actively involved with the health professionals as they review your case, see the list of Second Opinion

Centers provided in the resources section of this chapter or contact the Cancer Information Service at the national number, 1-800-4-CANCER.

While Second Opinion Centers are unique because they offer patients an unusual measure of involvement and participation in the review and analysis of the diagnosis, a sound second opinion or treatment for cancer can be obtained through many hospitals, oncology centers, and medical centers. In addition, hospitals with cancer programs approved by the American College of Surgeons offer tumor board meetings where your medical records can be reviewed by an objective, multidisciplinary panel of specialists.

American College of Surgeons Approved Cancer Programs

The American College of Surgeons maintains a state-by-state listing of all cancer programs that it approves. This free catalog is in the process of being updated to identify the hospital's cancer program category, such as "Comprehensive Cancer Program," "Teaching Hospital Cancer Program," "Community Hospital Comprehensive Cancer Program," "Community Hospital Cancer Program," "Hospital Associate Cancer Program," and "Special Cancer Program." The updated catalog also will include information about resources and services available at the hospitals that are oriented specifically to cancer patients.

The catalog is published annually and is available by calling 312-664-4050. See the resources section at the end of this chapter for more information about the catalog.

When the Doctors Disagree

Sometimes doctors will disagree on the diagnosis or proposed treatment. While it is unsettling to have medical experts disagree, it is vital for you to study the available options and talk about the treatment options with family, friends, support group members, and medical professionals.

You may want to have the medical specialists in disagreement provide their opinions written in simple, easy to understand language for your review. Also, you may need to realize that because medicine is an art, as well as a science, doctors do sometimes disagree on diagnoses or treatment options. Your responsibility is to make your best effort to select the treatment method and medical professional with whom you feel most able to communicate and who seems to make the most sense.

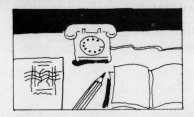

Resources for Getting a Second Opinion and Treatment

Information about obtaining a second opinion or treatment for cancer is available from the Cancer Information Service— 1-800-4-CANCER, your local office of the American Cancer Society, National Cancer Institute-designated Cancer Centers, Second Opinion Centers, and the American College of Surgeons.

Clinical Center of the National Institutes of Health

The Clinical Center of the National Institutes of Health provides medical care at no cost to patients providing they meet specific requirements of a particular research study. Patients must be referred by their physician and must have a diagnosis and complete medical history. Upon completion of the research study, patients are returned to the care of their referring physician.

For more information, or a pamphlet entitled, "Patient Admission Procedures," contact:

> The Director
> Clinical Center
> National Institutes of Health
> Building 10, Room 2C128
> Bethesda, Maryland 20892
>
> 301-496-4891 (Patient Referral Services)

National Cancer Institute-designated Cancer Centers

Cancer Centers listed below have passed a peer review board demonstrating high quality work in such areas as cancer research, prevention, detection, diagnosis, treatment, training, and education. They receive a government-funded Cancer Center Support Grant and the special identification as a National Cancer Institute-designated Cancer Center.

The National Cancer Institute-designated Cancer Centers listed below **entirely in bold face** show their designation as a Comprehensive Cancer Center. While all of the cancer centers in this list have passed the same rigorous peer review panel identifying them as excellent patient referral centers, the designation as Comprehensive is the responsibility of the National Cancer Advisory Board (NCAB). Approval by the NCAB is contingent on the center fulfilling the criteria of that Board.

The National Cancer Institute-designated Cancer Centers can provide second opinions, cancer treatment, and patient referral suggestions. The telephone numbers listed here are, for the most part, for the office that accepts calls from new patients seeking help. In a few instances, the telephone number is a switchboard. In either case, explain that you are a patient seeking information about possible treatment at that facility.

ALABAMA

**University of Alabama at Birmingham
Comprehensive Cancer Center
University Station
Birmingham, Alabama 35294
205-934-3690**

ARIZONA

Arizona Cancer Center
New Patient Referral
University of Arizona
College of Medicine
1501 North Campbell Avenue
Tucson, Arizona 85724
602-626-6372

CALIFORNIA

**Kenneth Norris Jr., Cancer Hospital
and Research Institute
University of Southern California
Patient/Physician Referral Office
P.O. Box 33804
1441 Eastlake Avenue
Los Angeles, California 90033-0804
213-226-2370**

**Jonsson Comprehensive Cancer Center
Patient Research Information and Referral Service
Louis Factor Health Sciences Building
UCLA Center for the Health Sciences
Los Angeles, California 90024
213-825-8727**

Northern California Cancer Center
1301 Shoreway Road, Suite 425
P.O. Box 2030
Belmont, California 94002-5030
415-591-4484
Ask for Pamela Priest

University of California at San Diego Cancer Center
UCSD Medical Center
225 Dickinson Street H-811 K
San Diego, California 92103
619-543-6178

Cancer Research Center
Beckman Research Institute
City of Hope
Patient Referral Office
1500 East Duarte Road
Duarte, California 91010
800-423-7119
800-535-1390 *(within California)*

CONNECTICUT

Yale University Comprehensive Cancer Center
School of Medicine
333 Cedar Street, Room 205 WWW
New Haven, Connecticut 06510
203-785-4095

DISTRICT OF COLUMBIA

Vincent T. Lombardi
Cancer Research Center
Georgetown University Medical Center
Division of Medical Oncology
3800 Reservoir Road, N.W.
Washington, D.C. 20007
202-625-7708

Howard University Cancer Center
Cancer Screening Clinic
2041 Georgia Avenue, N.W.
Washington, D.C. 20060
202-636-5665

FLORIDA

Papanicolaou Comprehensive Cancer Center
University of Miami Medical School
1475 N.W. 12th Avenue
P.O. Box 016960 (D8-4)
Miami, Florida 33101
305-548-4810

ILLINOIS

Illinois Cancer Council
36 South Wabash Avenue, Suite 700
Chicago, Illinois 60603
1-800-4-CANCER

A consortium composed of eight medical schools and other
agencies that have a significant interest in cancer.

Northwestern Medical Faculty Foundation
Medical Oncology
222 East Superior Street
Chicago, Illinois 60611
312-908-8697

The University of Chicago
Cancer Research Center
5841 South Maryland Avenue
Box 444
Chicago, Illinois 60637
312-702-6180

KENTUCKY

Lucille Parker Markey Cancer Center
University of Kentucky Medical Center
800 Rose Street
Lexington, Kentucky 40536-0093
606-257-4500

MARYLAND

Johns Hopkins Oncology Center
New Patient Coordinator
600 North Wolfe Street
Baltimore, Maryland 21205
301-955-8964

MASSACHUSETTS

Dana-Farber Cancer Institute
New Patient Referrals
44 Binney Street
Boston, Massachusetts 02115
617-732-3476

MICHIGAN

Meyer L. Prentis Comprehensive
  Cancer Center of Metropolitan Detroit
Oncology Clinic
110 East Warren Street
Detroit, Michigan 48201
313-745-4329

MINNESOTA

Mayo Clinic Comprehensive Cancer Center
Communications Coordinator
200 First Street, S.W.
Rochester, Minnesota 55905
507-284-3413

NEW HAMPSHIRE

Norris Cotton Cancer Center
Dartmouth-Hitchcock Medical Center
2 Maynard Street
Hanover, New Hampshire 03755
603-646-5527

NEW YORK

Memorial Sloan-Kettering Cancer Center
1275 York Avenue
New York, New York 10021
212-794-7722

Mt. Sinai Medical Center
Department of Neoplastic Diseases
#1 Gustave Levy Place
New York, New York 10029
212-650-6368

Note: Callers will need to leave their name and number with
     receptionist. A health professional will return the call.

Roswell Park Memorial Institute
666 Elm Street
Buffalo, New York 14263
716-845-2300

Cancer Research Center
Albert Einstein College of Medicine
Division of Medical Oncology
Montefiore Hospital and Medical Center
210th Street and Bainbridge Avenue
Bronx, New York 10467
212-430-4826

Columbia University Comprehensive Cancer Center
College of Physicians & Surgeons
Division of Medical Oncology
630 West 168th Street
New York, New York 10032
212-305-6730

Cancer Center
New York University Medical Center
Division of Oncology
550 First Avenue
New York, New York 10016
212-340-7227

University of Rochester Cancer Center
Box 704, 601 Elmwood Avenue
Rochester, New York 14642
716-275-4911

NORTH CAROLINA

Comprehensive Cancer Center
Duke University Medical Center
25178 Morris Building
P.O. Box 3814, Trent Avenue
Durham, North Carolina 27710
919-684-2282

Lineberger Cancer Research Center (237H)
School of Medicine
University of North Carolina at Chapel Hill
Chapel Hill, North Carolina 27514
919-966-3036

Oncology Research Center
Director's Office
Bowman Gray School of Medicine of
  Wake Forest University
300 South Hawthorne Road
Winston-Salem, North Carolina 27103
919-748-4464

OHIO

**Ohio State University Comprehensive
  Cancer Center
The Ohio State University Hospitals
410 West 10th Avenue
Columbus, Ohio 43210
614-421-8619**

PENNSYLVANIA

**Fox Chase/University of Pennsylvania
  Comprehensive Cancer Center**

**The Fox Chase Cancer Center
American Oncologic Hospital
New Patient Referral Office
Central and Shelmire Avenues
Philadelphia, Pennsylvania 19111
215-728-2570**

**University of Pennsylvania
  Cancer Center
7 Silverstein Pavillion
3400 Spruce Street
Philadelphia, Pennsylvania 19104
215-662-6334**

RHODE ISLAND

Brown University
Roger Williams Cancer Center
825 Chalkstone Avenue
Providence, Rhode Island 02908
401-456-2581

TENNESSEE

St. Jude Children's Research Hospital
332 North Lauderdale
Memphis, Tennessee 38101
901-522-0300

TEXAS

University of Texas System Cancer Center
M.D. Anderson Hospital & Tumor Institute
New Patient Referral Office
1515 Holcombe Boulevard
Houston, Texas 77030
713-792-6161
Note: Physician Referral Only

University of Texas Medical Branch
UTMB Cancer Center
4.160 John Sealy Hospital
Route E-65
Galveston, Texas 77550
409-761-1862

UTAH

Utah Regional Cancer Center
University of Utah Medical Center
50 North Medical Drive
Salt Lake City, Utah 84132
801-581-8793

VERMONT

Vermont Regional Cancer Center
University of Vermont
1 South Prospect Street
Burlington, Vermont 05401
802-656-4580

VIRGINIA

Massey Cancer Center
Medical College of Virginia
Virginia Commonwealth University
MCV Station, Box 37
Richmond, Virginia 23298
804-786-9992

WASHINGTON

Fred Hutchinson Cancer Research Center
1124 Columbia Street
Seattle, Washington 98104
206-467-5000
Note: This facility treats leukemia and related diseases only
      through bone marrow transplants.

WISCONSIN

University of Wisconsin Clinical Cancer Center
600 Highland Avenue
Madison, Wisconsin 53792
608-263-8600

Second Opinion Centers

Second Opinion Centers provide patients the opportunity to participate with a team of specialists to review their diagnosis, medical history, pathology reports, biopsy slides, and other facts to provide a sound second opinion about the best course of treatment. Pathologists, medical oncologists, radiologists, surgeons, and others are a part of the review meeting, along with the patients and their families.

Contact the Cancer Information Service by using the toll-free number—1-800-4-CANCER—or contact one of the Second Opinion Centers listed below. If you call one of the Second Opinion Centers, be sure to request the person listed as the contact.

ARIZONA

The University of Arizona Cancer Center
Arizona Health Sciences Center
Tucson, Arizona 85724
602-626-6372

Contact: Charlene Sass
Scheduling Time: Varies based on case; usually within one week
Requirements: Bring complete medical history, hospital discharge summaries, physician's notes, slides, scans, and x rays. For out-of-state patients, the initial contact should be made by the primary physician.
Additional Information: Serves patients eighteen and older.
Cost: $126 fee, plus any additional tests or doctors' services

ARKANSAS

St. Vincent Infirmary
St. Vincent Infirmary Cancer Center
2 St. Vincent Circle
Little Rock, Arkansas 72205
501-660-3900

Contact: April Johnson, Coordinator
Scheduling Time: Approximately ten days
Requirements: Need all records and reports forty-eight hours before panel meeting. Panel meets Wednesdays, 5-7 P.M.
Additional Information: Serves patients eighteen years of age or older.
Also offers a Stop Smoking Program, colorectal cancer screening, and breast cancer imaging programs.
Cost: No charge

CALIFORNIA

University of California, San Diego
University of California, San Diego Cancer Center
220 Dickinson Street
San Diego, California 92103
619-543-6187

Contact: Division of Hematology/Oncology Office
Scheduling Time: Usually seven to ten days
Requirements: Patients are responsible for bringing records and reports with them or sending them in advance.
Cost: Usually $120-$140 for any medical examinations that are needed

ILLINOIS

Northwestern Memorial Hospital
Member of The McGaw Medical Center
 of Northwestern University
Section of Hematology/Oncology
Superior Street and Fairbanks Court
Chicago, Illinois 60611
312-908-5284

Contact: All physicians listed below diagnose and treat all cancer diseases. Many physicians have a particular focus as indicated.
  Breast cancer and breast cancer screening: Sigmund Weitzman, M.D.
  Breast, melanoma, sarcoma: Jamie Von Roenn, M.D.
  Colon, rectal, gastric: Al Benson, M.D.
  Cutaneous T-cell lymphomas, lung cancer, biological response modifiers: Steven Rosen, M.D.
  General Hematology/Medical Oncology: John Merrill, M.D., and John Shaw, M.D., 312-908-7868
  Head, neck, breast cancer: Merrill Kies, M.D.
  Hematology clotting disorders: Hau Kwann, M.D.
  Hodgkin's disease, lymphomas, leukemia: Jane Winter, M.D.
  Hodgkin's disease, non-Hodgkin's disease, lymphomas, biological response modifiers, leukemia: Leo I. Gordon, M.D.
  Prostate, bladder, renal: Dennis Citrin, M.D.
Scheduling Time: Seven to ten days
Requirements: Send all medical records four to five days before meeting.
Additional Information: Serves patients sixteen and older.
Cost: To be determined; based on diagnosis and treatment

Loyola University Medical Center

2160 S. First Avenue
Maywood, Illinois 60153
312-531-3336

Contact: Richard Fisher, M.D.
Scheduling Time: Seven to ten days
Requirements: Patient can bring or send in advance all medical records.
Additional Information: Serves young adults and adults.
Cost: $200-$450

IOWA

University of Iowa Hospitals & Clinics

University of Iowa Cancer Center
Iowa City, Iowa 52242
319-335-7905

Contact: Cancer Center
Scheduling Time: Usually seven to fourteen days
Requirements: Bring all medical reports, x rays, slides, and scans or send them in advance.
Additional Information: Serves children as well as adults.
Cost: Approximately $100

MARYLAND

The Johns Hopkins Oncology Center

600 North Wolfe Street
Baltimore, Maryland 21205
301-955-8964

Contact: Peggy Anderson/Referral Coordinator
Scheduling Time: Within seven to fourteen days
Requirements: All medical records, pathology slides, x rays, and scans must be received by the center forty-eight hours in advance of the appointment.
Cost: $200 professional fee initial visit

MICHIGAN

The Meyer L. Prentis Comprehensive Cancer Center
University Health Center
4201 St. Antoine
Detroit, Michigan 48201

313-745-4700

Contact: Ms. MacKenzie
Scheduling Time: One day
Requirements: Patient needs to bring all available medical records or send them in advance.
Cost: $125

MISSOURI

R. A. Bloch Cancer Management Center
4410 Main Street
Kansas City, Missouri 64111

816-932-8453

Contact: Cancer Hot Line
Scheduling Time: Usually two weeks
Requirements: Patient is responsible for getting all medical records, x rays, scans, pathology slides, and reports, along with a summary letter from the physician. Patient and family are urged to meet with staff before the review board meeting and to participate in delivering records to board members. The staff prefers to accept patients who have not already had a second opinion consultation at a major cancer center. The Center usually limits service to residents of the states of Kansas and Missouri.

Additional Information: A psychologist participates in every board meeting and meets briefly with the patient and family immediately after the panel meeting.
Cost: No charge

NEW HAMPSHIRE

Norris Cotton Cancer Center
Dartmouth-Hitchcock Medical Center
2 Maynard Street
Hanover, New Hampshire 03756
603-646-5527

Contact: O. Ross McIntyre, M.D.
Scheduling Time: Within two weeks of request
Requirements: Medical reports, tests, and pathology reports should be made available several days before the meeting.
Cost: Hourly rate based on the number of specialists; probable total cost $300-$500

NEW YORK

Regional Cancer Center at Lourdes Hospital
169 Riverside Drive
Binghamton, New York 13905
607-798-5307

Contact: Medical Oncology Department
Scheduling Time: Two weeks
Requirements: Need complete set of patient's records including x-ray films and biopsy slides.
Cost: Varies based on number of specialists involved; approximately $300-$500

Montefiore Medical Center
111 East 210th Street
Bronx, New York 10467
212-920-4826

Contact: Department of Oncology, Peter H. Wiernik, M.D.
Scheduling Time: Usually within one week
Requirements: Send written reports seven days in advance, if possible.
Additional Information: Serves patients sixteen years of age and older.
Cost: $225

Roswell Park Memorial Institute

Buffalo, New York 14263

716-845-3385

Contact: Andrew A. Gage, M.D., Associate Institute Director for Clinical Affairs
Scheduling Time: Seven days
Requirements: Need patient's medical records one week before meeting.
Additional Information: Serves children, adolescents, and adults.
Cost: Varies with service; approximately $200

Mount Sinai Medical Center

The Associates of Neoplastic Diseases
19 East 98th Street, Suite 4A-F
New York, New York 10029

212-650-6368

Contact: The Associates of Neoplastic Diseases
Scheduling Time: Usually one to three weeks
Requirements: Bring all medical records to meeting.
Additional Information: Serves adults; contact Pediatrics for young patients.
Cost: $250

University of Rochester Cancer Center

Box 704
601 Elmwood Avenue
Rochester, New York 14642

716-275-4911; 800-462-6763 (toll-free in New York State only)

Contact: Assistant to the Director for Public Affairs
Scheduling Time: Minimum of ten to fourteen days
Requirements: Need all medical records and reports one week before meeting.
Costs: Varies

OHIO

University Hospitals
The Ireland Cancer Center
2074 Abington
Cleveland, Ohio 44106
216-844-8453

Contacts vary with specialty; see list below.
  Breast, colon, gastro-intestinal tumors: Thomas R. Spitzer, M.D., 216-844-8510
  Melanoma or skin cancer: David Bickers, M.D., 216-844-3177
  Pediatrics: Susan Shurin, M.D., 216-844-3345
  Head & neck: Lawrence T. Goodnough, M.D., 216-844-3162
  Neuro-Oncology: James S. Hewlett, M.D., 216-844-8547
  Leukemia, lung, lymphomas: Hillard M. Lazarus, M.D., 216-844-3629
  Gynecologic tumors: Michael S. Macfee, M.D., 216-844-3340
  Bone tumors: John Makley, M.D., 216-844-3033
  Bladder & prostate: Martin I. Resnick, M.D., 216-844-3009
  Other: Nathan A. Berger, M.D., 216-844-8453
Scheduling Time: Usually seven days
Requirements: Need case summary from physician, all pathology slides, x rays, and test results.
Additional Information: Serves children as well as adults.
Cost: Varies depending on case

Ohio State University Hospital
Room N1012B
Doan Hall
410 W. 10th Avenue
Columbus, Ohio 43210
614-293-8619

Contact: John Reed, Outpatient Coordinator, Division of Hematology/Oncology
Scheduling Time: Ten to thirty days
Requirements: Send all medical records fifteen to thirty days before meeting.
Additional Information: Serves patients eighteen and older.
Cost: To be determined

PENNSYLVANIA

The Fox Chase Cancer Center
American Oncologic Hospital
Central and Shelmire Avenues
Philadelphia, Pennsylvania 19111
215-728-2570

Contact: New Patient Referral Office
Scheduling Time: Approximately one week
Requirements: Varies according to diagnosis. May include sending copies of personal medical records, x-ray films, and pathology slides prior to the first scheduled appointment.
Additional Information: Center primarily serves patients eighteen years of age and older.
Cost: Varies depending on services provided

RHODE ISLAND

The Roger Williams Cancer Center
Brown University
825 Chalkstone Avenue
Providence, Rhode Island 02908
401-456-2581

Contact: Alan B. Weitberg, M.D.
Scheduling Time: Usually within seven days
Requirements: Need biospy slides, copies of x rays, reports, and medical history before meeting.
Additional information: Serves patients seventeen years of age or older.
Cost: No charge

TENNESSEE

St. Jude Children's Research Hospital
P.O. Box 318
Memphis, Tennessee 38101
901-522-0300

Contact: William Crist, M.D.
Scheduling Time: Varies, usually seven days
Requirements: Patient or family may initiate contact, but physician referral required. Need medical records and reports (or summary of reports) and pathology slides of biopsy.
Additional Information: Majority of inquiries are handled via telephone. Some are done with patient present at review board meeting.
Cost: No charge

TEXAS

University of Texas Medical Branch
UTMB Cancer Center
4.160 JSH
Galveston, Texas 77550
409-761-1862

Contact: John Costanzi, M.D.
Scheduling Time: Usually one to two weeks
Requirements: Need all medical records and reports four to five days in advance.
Additional Information: Serves patients sixteen years of age or older.
Cost: Varies; approximately $75

WISCONSIN

University of Wisconsin Clinical Cancer Center
600 Highland Avenue
Madison, Wisconsin 53792
608-263-8600

Contact: Donald Trump, M.D.
Scheduling Time: Usually twenty-four to thirty-six hours
Requirements: Patients need to bring all medical records with them.
Additional Information: Serves adults primarily.
Cost: Approximately $250-300

American College of Surgeons Approved Cancer Programs

American College of Surgeons
Cancer Department
55 East Erie
Chicago, Illinois 60611
312-664-4050

The American College of Surgeons provides a catalog, available free of charge, which lists all of the approved cancer treatment programs in every state. The catalog is in the process of being updated in order to designate for each hospital the category of its cancer treatment program and provide information about the hospital's resources specifically available for cancer patients. The catalog is published annually.

Booklets

"Thinking of Having Surgery: Think About Getting a Second Opinion." Available free from the Consumer Information Center, Department 601-P, Pueblo, Colorado 81009; 303-948-3334.

A one-page pamphlet that discusses the value of a second opinion for non-emergency surgery, presents questions to ask about the proposed operation, offers suggestions for when a second opinion is useful, and provides ideas, including a toll-free number (1-800-638-6833) for locating a physician in your area to give a second opinion.

CHAPTER THREE

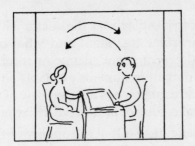

Communicating with Your Doctor

One of the most important things patients can do during the critical months of stabilizing and regaining their health is to communicate effectively with their doctors. Open and honest communication with health care professionals is vital to establishing a climate of trust and mutual respect, which can foster healing and renewal. Open communication allows both the patient and the physician to understand that they are working as equal team members on the very important project of beating back the progress of the disease.

Open communication is also valuable because it permits trust and confidence to develop between patient and doctor, allowing the patient to have confidence that the physician's prescribed treatment will work.

Many of us were brought up to accept whatever an authority figure told us. We were discouraged from asking questions or from challenging authority. When you are the patient and your life is at stake, the best policy is to *ask* questions and *question* authority. Patients who participate actively in their recovery need to feel free to ask questions of their doctors. Patients need to be able to speak up if something the doctor says or does isn't clear or if some aspect of the doctor's language, diagnosis, or treatment needs an explanation.

Patients need to be able to ask the doctor why he or she is recommending a particular treatment and what other options are available besides the recommended one. An informed patient who is aware of the variety of treatments available and their particular advantages or disadvantages has a larger view of the solutions and is better able to take control and make an informed decision.

Sometimes patients fear that the quality of their care will deteriorate if they ask the doctor for detailed explanations or question the doctor about decisions or recommendations. Patients need to work through that roadblock and come to realize that well-informed patients who require thorough explanations will receive the same or better quality care as any other patient.

Patients also need to recognize the choices they have—both to seek other doctors' opinions to substantiate their doctor's recommendations and to change doctors if necessary. Time is a precious commodity when a patient is beginning the fight against cancer, yet the time spent seeking a second or third opinion is well spent if it leads to an informed decision to select the doctor or the treatment program that seems best.

What follows are a few basic guidelines for communicating effectively with your doctor.

It's the Questions That Count

Be prepared in advance with the list of questions (and follow-up questions) you want to discuss with your doctor. Keep your list handy when you visit the doctor's office or when you are expecting a call. You will be more satisfied with the exchange if you think through your questions, wildest fears, and concerns in advance, so you can clearly and concisely explain your problems and listen intently to the doctor's response.

Richard Bloch, lung cancer survivor and Honorary Chairman of H&R Block, Inc., encourages patients to ask their doctor specific questions about side effects of their treatment. "An important one," Bloch states, "is 'Which side effects, in your opinion, should I expect?' " Bloch reminds patients that "doctors are required to tell all possible side effects of the treatment and this list can scare anyone out of their mind. The best solution to this dilemma," Bloch adds, "is, after listening to the list, to ask 'Which of those I might expect to occur?' "

They Won't Know Unless You Tell Them

Be willing to give your doctor as much information as you can about yourself and the special needs or attention you may be requesting. Many times this frankness and openness will bridge what, at first, seems like a communication gap.

For example, my oncologist tells the story of some of his patients (and I include myself in this group), who are clearly disappointed when he calls to say something like, "Your test results are good." Such patients, he explains, want stronger reassurance and more positive language, so when he calls them he says, "Your tests are great," or "Your tests are perfect." (Once, when he called me to say "Your test results are better than ever," I made him take time to explain how this could possibly be, since he had been describing them as "great" all along. Useful information about the tests came from that discussion.) Test results may well just be test results, but if subtleties in the doctors' language are important, let them know.

Recognizing the Doctor's Position

Patients place especially high demands on their doctors and have exceedingly rigorous expectations for the quality of treatment they provide as well. While it is important to communicate clearly with the doctor and to be sure that he or she understands our particular needs, we need to remember that our doctors are working with many other patients, as well. Some of these other patients may be much less healthy than we are.

The burden on health professionals working with patients who are chronically and seriously ill is a heavy one. That burden may make the doctor seem distant, unsympathetic, removed, or uncaring at times. We feel we need the doctor's attention just when his or her energy and primary concern is with another, more needy patient. Also, some doctors protect themselves from pain and loss by not letting themselves get close to any patient.

It is fair for us to give doctors with whom we are experiencing difficulty in communicating some extra time before we give up on them as somehow just "not right" for us. It may be that after two or three appointments, we can come to see that the doctor is caring and open to our particular needs.

It is worth remembering that doctors who are very skillful may not happen to be as outgoing or demonstrative as we might wish. Even though they may be reserved or even gruff, doctors who listen with respect and communicate honestly are worth investing the effort in to learn to work with successfully.

Switch—When All Else Fails

If you have decided that you do not feel at ease getting treatment or information from your surgeon, radiologist, or oncologist, and you cannot make any progress toward achieving that comfort, speak openly to the doctor about it. If a frank discussion with your doctor doesn't make an impact on his or her behavior, be open to the necessity of finding another doctor who can meet your needs better. You may find that one of the other doctors in the same office or hospital department matches your style better. Talk with friends, members of your support group, or your family physician for suggestions.

Don't be ashamed or frightened to switch doctors to find one with whom you are more comfortable. My first months fighting cancer, I saw a specialist who is widely recognized as one of the best in his field. But seeing him was a difficult experience. Because of his reputation, the office was filled with patients. Waiting time varied, but was always one hour and many times two hours or more. Meetings with him were limited, tense sessions, often interrupted by telephone calls or queries from the receptionist.

I was reluctant to leave his care for fear that continuity in my treatment would suffer. When I shared my dilemma with my counselor, he reminded me that all doctors rely on the patient's chart, test results, and other documents in the file to refresh their memory of the case and that changing doctors would not set my recovery back.

That reminder enabled me to switch to a different specialist in the same office—to a doctor who had access to the same research insights, who had an appreciation for my needs, and who had a caring and concerned manner. Immediately, my feelings about office visits changed dramatically. Time with the doctor was efficient, but unharried, as he gave careful attention to my questions and responded with thoughtful, detailed answers.

While no one would encourage a patient to change doctors casually, patients need to be prepared to recognize those times when they can make a significant improvement in their satisfaction with the health care they are receiving by opting for a change.

Your family physician, or primary care physician, can be a valuable resource in selecting a different specialist. Other valuable resources are a local hospital with a cancer program approved by the American College of Surgeons, the Cancer Information Service (CIS), your local American Cancer Society Office, National Cancer Institute-designated Cancer Centers, or members of your support group.

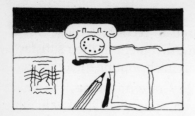

Resources for Communicating with Your Doctor

Books

The Road Back to Health: Coping With the Emotional Side of Cancer,
Neil A. Fiore, Bantam, 1986.

In *The Road Back to Health,* Neil Fiore, a psychologist and cancer patient, gives valuable advice about being an active patient, finding doctors who suit your needs, and learning how to participate with your doctors in your treatment.

Chapter Three, "Becoming an Active Patient," includes discussions such as "There is More to You Than Cancer," "Who Knows What's Best for You?" and "The Patient as Expert." In Chapter Four, "You and Your Doctor," discusses useful information such as "How to Find a Good Doctor," "Realistic Trust or Blind Faith," "Shared Responsibility, Shared Authority," and "Asking Questions."

Booklets

"Communication Between You, the Cancer Patient, and Your Doctor—A Conversation with a Doctor Who is Also a Cancer Patient." To request this free publication, call 305-548-4821, or write Cancer Information Service, P.O. Box 016960 (D8-4), Miami, Florida 33101. Copies are limited. Generally, individual copies are sent free of charge. Requests for quantities over five are charged at $1 per copy.

This brochure, in a question-and-answer format, covers such issues as, "When I am given a different opinion from two or more doctors, what should I do?"; "How do I get a second opinion without offending the first doctor?"; "How do I know

I am getting a good doctor?"; "How can I tactfully confront my doctor with the fact that I don't feel we are communicating effectively?"; "How do I register a complaint about my doctor?"; "How can I get compassionate concern from my doctor?" An introduction to the brochure describes the role of the oncologist and the value of a solid relationship between the patient and oncologist.

"Talking With Your Doctor," American Cancer Society, Publication #4636. 1987.

This easy to read pamphlet provides helpful discussions to assist patients in establishing on-going, satisfying communications with their doctors. Topics focus on issues such as "Ask Yourself 'How Much Do I Need to Know?' ", "Understanding Your Doctor," "Working on a Dialogue," "Changes in the Relationship," and "When Is the Best Time to Call if You Have a Question?"

"Taking Time: Support for People With Cancer and the People Who Care About Them," National Cancer Institute, Bethesda, Maryland 20892, 1983.

The chapter entitled "When You Need Assistance" describes the importance of working as a team with your health professionals, the value of raising questions with your doctor, and the appropriateness of changing doctors when an open, trusting relationship cannot be established.

CHAPTER FOUR

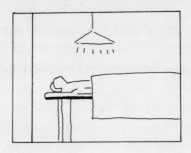

Surgery

Going into the hospital for surgery is scary. With some advance preparation and an understanding of what is going to happen, you can learn what to expect from surgery and recovery and feel that you have more control over them. Here are a few suggestions for helping to prepare yourself for your hospital experience.

Interviewing the Surgeon

Ask your surgeon a variety of questions to help you know what to expect. These might include:

- ☐ Where he or she practices and what the hospital is like—small and friendly, a businesslike teaching and research facility, or a large but efficient hospital. Does the doctor practice in more than one hospital, one of which may be superior for this particular operation or in some other important way.
- ☐ How long the surgery will take.
- ☐ Whether general or local anesthesia will be required.

☐ How long after the operation you will be getting out of bed.

☐ How long you will be in the hospital.

☐ When you can expect to return to your regular responsiblities, either part-time or full-time.

☐ What kind of discomfort, if any, you can expect after surgery.

☐ Where any scars will be and what they will look like.

☐ Whether the surgery normally results in any short- or long-term sensations, such as numbness, twinges, or pain.

☐ Whether the surgery can be handled on an in-and-out rather than an inpatient basis.

☐ Which anesthesiologist the doctor prefers to work with.

☐ What the costs of the suggested surgery and any follow-up treatment will be.

Setting the Most Convenient Schedule

Work with your surgeon's office assistant to schedule the surgery promptly but at a convenient time. For example, biopsies scheduled on a Friday may require very little time away from work. However, because pathology departments do not work on weekends, biopsies scheduled on Friday mean two additional days of waiting for the results. If scheduling is important, consider it carefully before agreeing to a date.

If you are having in-and-out surgery, be sure to have someone accompany you or scheduled to pick you up after the surgery. If you are scheduled for inpatient surgery, ask if there is any way you can avoid an additional night in the hospital by doing routine tests a day or two before the surgery (on an outpatient basis) and arriving early in the morning on the day of surgery.

Interviewing the Anesthesiologist

If you are having a general anesthesia and the hospital you are using is large enough to offer a choice of anesthesiologists, request names from either the surgeon or his or her office assistants. Ask for names of one or two anesthesiologists with whom the doctor prefers to work. Call the anesthesiologists immediately to screen them.

When you speak with the anesthesiologists, try to get a sense of your rapport with them. Ask them about their credentials, how long they have been practicing, and what hospitals they use. Ask them to explain what they will be doing during the surgery and why. If you have had any particular reaction from anesthesia in the past or have any other special condition, be sure to mention it. Ask them about costs you can anticipate for their services.

Using Relaxation Responses

While you are in the hospital awaiting surgery, use relaxation response techniques to keep as calm and relaxed as possible. If you have an inexpensive tape player, listen to relaxing environmental sounds, music, or suggestions for relaxation responses.

If you don't have tapes or a tape player available, gently close your eyes and begin to inhale and exhale deeply and fully. Picture youself at your most favorite quiet place and concentrate on relaxing every muscle in your body. Start at your head and move the relaxation throughout your body, from the muscles in your head and face to your neck and chest, arms and hands, trunk, hips, knees, legs, and feet. Breathe deeply and think the words, "Relax and be calm," as you focus on relaxing your body and your mind.

Learning the Routine

Ask the hospital floor nurses what the typical procedure and routines are before and after surgery. Start with the basic questions every good reporter uses to get the complete picture—what happens, when, where, why, and how. Knowing these things will give you a clearer picture and a feeling of better control.

With my three surgeries for cancer in the same hospital within a seven-month period, I became quite familiar with its procedures. Gradually, I learned more and more about the routine by experiencing it first-hand. Understandably enough, each surgery became significantly easier to anticipate and recover from because of my familiarity with the experiences. I recommend getting this information more efficiently than I did—talk with the nurses throughout your stay about what you can expect to happen.

Taking Time for Yourself

If you have time before surgery, get up and treat yourself to a relaxing, warm shower and shampoo. It may have to last you for a number of days because stitches from incisions need to be kept dry. Doctors will recommend only a sponge bath when you feel well enough for bathing.

I recommend time before surgery to be by yourself to reread favorite inspirational messages, to meditate on dynamic, fulfilling thoughts, and to reflect on favorite memories and relaxing scenes. Put yourself as much as possible, physically and mentally, in a frame of mind that is in charge of wonderfully fulfilling experiences. Imagine yourself after the surgery as healthy, renewed, and invigorated.

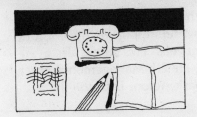

Resources for Preparing for Surgery

Bring an inexpensive tape player to the hospital along with some of your most soothing and relaxing music tapes, or try some of the relaxation tapes that follow.

"Environments: The Magic of Psycho-Acoustic Sound." Tapes in the series include "Slow Ocean," "English Meadows," "Sailboat," "Ultimate Thunderstorm," "Sounds of the Surf," "Canoe to Loon Lake," "Sailboat to Hidden Cove," "Redwood Forest Trail," "Storm on Wilderness Lake," "Tradewind Islands," and others. Available from The Nature Company, the tapes are $8.98 each. Telephone orders are accepted twenty-four hours a day at 800-227-1114.

"Suggestions for General Relaxation," by Lynn Brallier, is an introductory guide to relaxation. This tape, a powerful tool for relaxing the body and the mind, is used as a learning resource for individuals needing to manage stress and as a recovery aid in many hospitals and clinics throughout the country. The tape is available for $10.95* from the Stress/Health Management Center, 621 Maryland Avenue, N.E., Washington, D.C. 20002.

"Suggestions for Restful Sleep," by Lynn Brallier, is a soothing tape that allows the body and mind to let go of tension and drift into a restful sleep. Available from the Stress/Health Management Center, 621 Maryland Avenue, N.E., Washington, D.C. 20002, this tape is $10.95*.

"Relaxation and Imagery for the Person with Cancer," by Lynn Brallier, helps persons with cancer to relax, restore their energy, and build a positive base for gaining control of their experience with cancer. The tape helps develop methods and imagery for deep relaxation, which may enhance the effectiveness of medical procedures while supporting the immune system's battle against the cancer cells. This tape is also available for $10.95* from the Stress/Health Management Center, 621 Maryland Avenue N.E., Washington, D.C. 20002.

---

*All tapes by Lynn Brallier from the Stress/Health Mangement Center are $10.95, except for a special price of $20.95 for the purchase of "Suggestions for General Relaxation" and one other tape. Add $1.00 for postage and handling for the first tape and $.50 for each additional tape.

CHAPTER FIVE

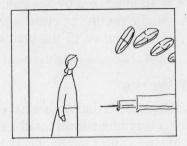

Chemotherapy

Many treatments for cancer will include a course of chemotherapy instead of, or in addition to, surgery or radiation therapy. The medical doctor who provides this treatment is an oncologist, one who specializes in the diagnosis and treatment of cancer. Oncologists can be medical oncologists, surgical oncologists, or radiation oncologists. Your surgeon or family doctor will recommend an oncologist.

Chemotherapy is a method of treating cancer through the use of drugs or medications. The anticancer drugs disrupt the ability of the cancer cells to grow and multiply.

When a group of chemotherapy drugs is used together to fight cancer, the process is called combination chemotherapy. When anticancer drugs are used after another treatment, such as surgery or radiation, to destroy any possible remaining cells, the process is called adjuvant chemotherapy.

Chemotherapy may be given in several ways, depending on the type of cancer and the drugs being used. The anticancer drugs may be taken orally, injected into a muscle, or injected or infused into a vein.

Chemotherapy is administered by the medical oncologist or oncology nurse. A specific routine or cycle is established which usually continues for the duration of the treatment specified by the oncologist.

Here's How It Works

It is useful to know that medical oncologists have their practices in a variety of locations, everywhere from small, private medical offices and hospitals to large cancer treatment centers. If you have a preference for one kind of environment, ask your medical oncologist if she or he practices in the type of location you prefer. You might ask your surgeon at the start to recommend a medical oncologist who practices in surroundings you find comfortable and reassuring.

Realize that the day of the week for your first visit to the medical oncologist for chemotherapy will most likely be the day for all your subsequent appointments. Think in advance about the schedule you prefer. Some patients prefer late afternoon appointments on a Friday so that no work time is spent recuperating from side effects. Some patients prefer their treatments early Monday morning so they can be finished with their chemotherapy early in the week.

Your visit to the medical oncologist will involve more than the chemotherapy treatment itself. In addition to periodic mini-physical exams, every visit will require that you have your finger pricked for immediate analysis of several drops of blood. This will allow a technician to count your white blood cells and determine if your white blood count is within the normal range. If there are occasions when your white blood count is below normal, the chemotherapy treatment will be postponed for several days to allow your white cells to rebuild.

An Important New Test

Every six weeks or so, your medical oncologist may take a sample of blood from your vein to track a variety of the body's functions. Some physicians are also requesting that a Carcino Embryonic Antigen (CEA) test be performed on the blood sample along with the other tests. This new test provides a basic analysis of the body's major functions to determine if there is any cellular activity in the body that shows rapid and uncontrolled growth or division.

Fighting Infections While on Chemotherapy

Because chemotherapy reduces the white blood cell count in the body, the system is more susceptible to infection. While you are going through chemotherapy treatments, be sure to notify your medical oncologist before you have dental work performed. This way he or she can check your white blood cell count to be sure that it is high enough to fight any bacteria that may enter the blood stream from the mouth during the dental work.

It is generally best to have teeth cleaning or other periodontal work done right before the next chemotherapy treatment, so that the white blood cells are at their greatest number. If this timing is not possible or if your white blood cell count is low for other reasons, the oncologist can prescribe antibiotics to control any infection that may arise from the dental work.

Patients with replacement heart valves have antibiotics prescribed for them during chemotherapy as a matter of course to fight off any infections that may occur.

Chemotherapy and Hair Loss

Hair may drop out because hair follicles are highly sensitive to the massive doses of drugs. If hair does react, it will take several weeks after starting chemotherapy for the impact of the drugs to affect the hair.

If your doctor offers it and recommends that it may help, you can use an "ice cap" or "cold cap" for twenty minutes before, during, and for twenty minutes after your chemotherapy injection. This "ice cap," an icy headdress you put on your head to chill the scalp, may help reduce hair loss in some chemotherapy situations.

If your hair is thin or the doctor anticipates that your hair loss will be quite significant, get a wig or hairpiece from a wig shop or department store before you lose any hair. Some hospitals, cancer centers, or offices of the American Cancer Society may provide wigs or hairpieces. Have your hair clipped short to make it easier and cooler to wear your wig. You may want to get a sleeping cap for bedtime. Remember that your hair will grow back as soon as the massive doses of drugs are reduced.

Whether you lose some or all of your hair during chemotherapy treatments, be sure to take especially good care of your hair and scalp during this time. Use gentle shampoos, soft brushes, and low heat when drying or curling hair. Postpone dyeing your hair, getting a permanent, or using any other harsh chemicals on it until chemotherapy treatments are finished. It is also recommended to avoid braids, cornrows, naturals, or sleeping on rollers.

Planning a Spirit Booster

While some patients on chemotherapy report no adverse side effects, many people find it necessary to stay at home and rest for a day shortly after their chemotherapy treatments. Reactions from one treatment to the next seem to be fairly consistent. Reactions don't seem to build up over the months and become considerably worse.

If you find you need a day or more after your chemotherapy treatment to recuperate, schedule something that perks up your spirits for the first moments you feel you can get out of bed. Even if you aren't feeling 100 percent great, having a favorite spot to visit, a short trip out with a special friend, an excursion to see a funny movie, or another enjoyable pastime seems to speed up the recovery process. For example, I had a standing appointment the day after chemotherapy treatments with my friend and hair stylist to have my slightly-thinning hair styled. After that, I went for an hour's practice in conversational Italian with a tutor. I didn't learn a lot of Italian and sometimes I felt pretty shaky about being up, but both of these pre-planned events motivated me to get up and get going with something fun.

Chemotherapy and That Queasy Feeling

Be aware that during the course of your chemotherapy treatment—including the days between when you're not taking any chemotherapy treatments—you may have a general uneasy, queasy feeling. Some women have mentioned that it reminds them of morning sickness. This queasy feeling may be heightened by riding in a car, train, plane, or elevator. While this is a minor nuisance, you may ask your doctor to recommend ways to control it. Some persons have found that aerobic exercise is effective in reducing this queasy feeling.

If you have significant trouble with nausea, consider asking your physician or medical oncologist for medication to help control it. You will need to experiment to find the best drug and dosage for your own body. The medication, whether injected or taken orally, acts to control the nausea by numbing the portion of the brain that controls nausea. Thus, the medication usually entails such side effects as grogginess or sleepiness.

If you live alone and do not have the strength to cook or find the smells associated with preparing food distasteful or upsetting, check your local telephone directory or ask your doctor, American Cancer Society, Cancer Information Service, or the National Association of Meal Programs in Washington, D.C., for information about Meals on Wheels or Mobile Meals. This community service group delivers meals to the homes of the sick, disabled, frail, those over fifty years of age, or others.

Publications that focus specifically on nutrition during chemotherapy are available through the Cancer Information Service and your local American Cancer Society office. See the resources section of this chapter for more information.

Tastes, Smells, and That Queasy Feeling

Be prepared to have foods taste different during the time you're having chemotherapy treatments. Even your favorite foods may be distasteful. Most likely you will discover new foods that become your favorite or "security foods" while you're on chemotherapy. You may put aside some foods completely or at least until the chemo is over. I banished chocolate, barbecued foods, and mixtures with mayonnaise as being "unappetizing" for the time I was on chemotherapy.

In addition to being sensitive to certain tastes, you may find yourself more sensitive to and upset by certain smells. Certain fragrances from cosmetics, hand and body creams, and soaps, or stronger smells from dry-cleaned clothes or the barbecue grill can be upsetting.

Keeping the Fluids Moving

Drink significant amounts of fluids daily during the chemotherapy regimen. Some doctors recommend six to eight large glasses or approximately half a gallon. The water, juices, and soft drinks help keep the body fluids fresh and moving, so that no build-up of harmful chemicals can affect the body adversely. Alcoholic beverages are *not* to be used for fluids.

Taking the Chemotherapy Pills

Many individuals on chemotherapy take as few as one or as many as six pills for chemotherapy each day during the course of their treatment. You may find it useful to develop a system for taking the pills. For example, some people use a daily chart to check off the pills they have taken. Others find it useful to sort pills regularly into pill keepers, so the pills are readily available. I asked my best friend and roommate to be responsible for fixing the water glass and doling out the pill dosage each evening at an agreed-on time. Just being relieved of that task was for me a tremendous relief.

As a practical note, I suggest buying an inexpensive glass or cup to use regularly for taking the pills. When chemotherapy is over, get rid of the glass—you'll never need it again. Before I followed this method of having just one glass for taking the pills, I found I would not reuse any of the glasses again for a snack or meal. I had somehow shifted my feelings about chemotherapy pill-taking onto the glasses themselves.

Using a Role Model for Inspiration

Chemotherapy can be a grueling time—even when the treatment proceeds remarkably well and on schedule. Administering massive doses of drugs to the body takes its toll even in small ways: increased fatigue, frustration from being somewhat locked into fixed treatment schedules, anxiety that can accompany the treatment, and time spent waiting in doctors' offices.

I recommend focusing on a figure or symbol to be a constant reminder of the spirit of strength and self-sufficiency that chemotherapy asks of you. For example, I found a postcard of a pioneer who had a roughly-lettered sign on the back of all his worldly belongings that read "Oregon or Bust." The picture of that pioneer crystallized for me the spirit of determination that I needed for making the chemotherapy trek. I displayed that postcard prominently in my room, so that I could have before me a reminder that all of us can get through rough times to arrive at our promised land.

I destroyed the "Oregon or Bust" postcard when chemotherapy was over, because it had served its usefulness during hard times. A new, gentler response was in order after the chemotherapy—one that focused more on growth and increased coping than survival. The most important reason for destroying the card, of course, is because I don't intend to need it ever again.

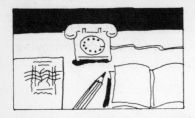

Resources about Chemotherapy

Books

Coping With Chemotherapy, Nancy Bruning, Ballantine Books, New York, 1986, $3.95. This book describes the various treatment options for cancer and, in particular, how chemotherapy works. Attention is given to how to decide if chemotherapy is right for a particular situation. The book offers coping suggestions for the mind, body, and spirit and examines the doctor-patient relationship. *Coping With Chemotherapy* includes a glossary of chemotherapy drugs, what they do, and what side effects they may cause.

Booklets

"Chemotherapy and You: A Guide to Self-Help During Treatment," NIH Publication No. 85-1136. National Cancer Institute, Bethesda, Maryland 20892.

This booklet gives a thorough, but easy to read, explanation of what chemotherapy is, how the treatment is given, the importance of diet during treatment and some of the common side effects. The most used anticancer drugs are described in detail along with how they are administered and any side effects that may be expected.

"What Is Chemotherapy?," American Cancer Society publication.

A one-page pamphlet that explains what chemotherapy is, how it is used and administered, and what its effects are. Precautions are suggested as well as valuable questions to discuss with your physician. Contact your local American Cancer Society office for a copy.

"Eating Hints: Recipes and Tips for Better Nutrition During Cancer Treatment," NIH Publication No. 84-2079. National Cancer Institute, Bethesda, Maryland 20892.

A spiral-bound booklet that offers easy-to-prepare recipes as well as practical information and advice for eating well during cancer treatment. The booklet is based on patient interviews and lists numerous suggestions to cope with particular problems, including nausea and vomiting, loss of appetite, mouth soreness or dryness, feeling tired, and intestinal upset. "Eating Hints" gives tips for adding protein and calories to meals and suggests options for patients needing soft food or food that is low in fat or fiber. Main dish, sauce and gravy, and dessert recipes are included to address the particular problems of cancer patients. The recipes are specifically created to be nutritious, easy to make, and tasty for the entire family.

Tapes

"Relaxation and Imagery for the Person with Cancer," by Lynn Brallier, helps persons with cancer to relax, restore their energy, and build a positive base for gaining control of their experience with cancer. The tape helps develop methods and imagery for deep relaxation, which may enhance the effectiveness of medical procedures while supporting the immune system's battle against the cancer cells. This audio tape is available for $10.95 from the Stress/Health Management Center, 621 Maryland Avenue N.E., Washington, D.C. 20002.

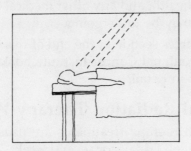

Radiation Therapy

Treatments for cancer may use radiation therapy instead of, or in addition to, surgery and chemotherapy. The medical professionals who provide this treatment are radiation therapists (or radiation oncologists), who are physicians who head a team made up of a radiation therapy nurse, a radiation therapy technologist (who delivers the treatment to the patient), and a radiation physicist (who determines the proper dose of radiation and checks that the machines deliver each dosage accurately). Your surgeon or family doctor will recommend a radiation therapist.

Radiation therapy consists of administering radiation externally or by implanting radiation temporarily or sometimes permanently into the body. This therapy involves using high-level doses of radiation to shrink a tumor or to stop the growth of cancerous cells by destroying them. External radiation therapy uses machines to direct the high-energy rays to the cancer and surrounding tissue. Internal radiation therapy consists of surgery (requiring either a local or general anesthesia) to place the radioactive materials—such as seeds, needles, wires, capsules, or wax molds—directly into the tumor or the surrounding body cavity.

A person's radiation therapy is individually determined for him or her and is based on the size and location of the tumor, the patient's general health, and any other medical treatment the patient has had or may be undergoing.

See the resources section at the end of this chapter for information about a National Cancer Institute booklet that describes radiation therapy in detail.

How External Radiation Therapy Works

External radiation therapy treatments are usually given once a day, Monday through Friday, for several weeks. The weekend rest periods give the healthy cells time to rebuild. While the dose of radiation may last only several minutes, the visit for radiation therapy may require thirty minutes or more for changing clothes and being positioned correctly under the equipment.

The first visit to the radiation therapist will most likely not involve a treatment. Instead, the radiation therapist will use x rays and other tests to do a "simulation" to locate the exact area of the body to receive the radiation rays. The radiation technologist will mark that exact place on the skin with indelible ink to outline the treatment area. The ink markings will probably remain throughout the treatment period, but notify your doctor if, for some reason, they should become faint during the course of treatment.

Radiation therapy treatments require that the patient sit or lie very still beneath the radiation equipment to ensure that only the specified location receives the treatment. After the machine is moved into place, the radiation technologist leaves the room and operates the equipment from a distant room connected to the treatment room via intercom, TV screen, or windows.

It is normal for patients to feel overwhelmed or fearful during their first experience with the radiation equipment. This is especially true when the patient is left alone in the room with the enormous equipment hovering above. It is natural to have fears and anxiety about the experience, especially at the beginning of the treatment program.

How Internal Radiation Therapy Works

Internal radiation therapy requires hospitalization for placing the radioactive material in the body and for several days while the implant is in place. Some hospitals may require a private room for the patient receiving a temporary radiation implant. Permanent implants usually require isolation in the hospital for several days until the strength of the radiation in the permanent implant is weaker and the patient can be discharged.

Because radiation from a temporary or permanent implant may expose others to high levels of radiation unnecessarily, health professionals will not spend much time in the room or near the bed. Visitors will be allowed in the room briefly each day if they maintain a safe distance of five feet or more. Many hospitals will not admit visitors under eighteen or women who are pregnant.

Radiation Therapy and Fatigue

The stress of treatment visits and the effects of radiation on healthy cells may cause a general feeling of fatigue or weariness. Naps, extra sleep at night, or an effort to cut back on physically demanding work and family or social responsibilities may help restore strength during the period of external radiation therapy.

Radiation Therapy and That Queasy Feeling

A feeling of nausea or loss of appetite is another reaction that sometimes occurs with external radiation therapy. Because eating well is so important during treatment for cancer, it is essential to find ways to keep nutritional intake up to par.

Some patients who experience nausea during their radiation treatment recommend eating a solid meal before the treatment to help calm the stomach and reduce nausea.

Some patients find snacking on small, frequent meals throughout the day and evening more successful than sitting down to three substantial meals each day. Other patients recommend determining several nutritious "security" foods that can be eaten easily and frequently during the days of radiation therapy and using these security foods as a base around which to build a meal.

If you live alone or do not have the strength to cook or find the smells associated with preparing food distasteful or upsetting, check your local telephone directory or ask your doctor, American Cancer Society, Cancer Information Service, or National Association of Meal Programs in Washington, D.C., for information about assistance from Meals on Wheels or Mobile Meals. This community service group delivers meals to the homes of the sick, disabled, frail, those over fifty years of age, or others.

Radiation Therapy and Skin Care

Most patients notice that their skin becomes dry and itchy in the treatment area. Because lotions or creams or petroleum jelly can interfere with the radiation therapy, be sure to follow advice from your radiation therapist about what to use to relieve this annoyance. The itchy, dry skin will clear up shortly after the completion of radiation therapy.

Some patients notice that their skin color in the treatment area discolors slightly and becomes somewhat darker. Usually this slight discoloration is permanent.

It is important for individuals going through radiation therapy to keep the sun from coming in contact with their skin. Long sleeves, hats with wide, floppy brims, and sunscreen lotions (with your doctor's approval) will help.

If your skin cracks or blisters, be sure to tell your doctor at once. This might require a change in treatment.

Radiation Therapy and Hair Loss

Some or all of the hair in the treatment area may drop out because of the radiation therapy. Usually this hair grows back after the treatments are completed.

If your hair is thin or the doctor anticipates that your hair loss will be significant, get a wig or hairpiece from a wig shop or department store before you lose any hair. Some hospitals, cancer centers, or offices of the American Cancer Society may provide wigs. Have your hair clipped short to make it easier and cooler to wear your wig. You may want to get a sleeping cap for bedtime.

Whether you lose some or all of your hair during radiation treatments, be sure to take especially good care of your hair and scalp during this time. Use gentle shampoos, soft brushes, and low heat when drying or curling hair. Postpone dyeing your hair, getting a permanent, or using any other harsh chemicals on your hair until radiation treatments are finished. It is also recommended to avoid braids, cornrows, naturals, or sleeping on rollers.

Planning a Spirit Booster

Remember that with some attention and a little advance planning your daily radiation treatment can be a positive experience.

Take along motivating, inspiring, or humorous readings to boost your spirits during the wait for radiation treatment. If you keep a journal of humorous personal events or a collection of your favorite cartoons, you may want to read through these.

Ask a friend or family member whose company you enjoy to accompany you for treatment. Just knowing that you have someone supportive with you can be a tremendous boost.

Think about very positive outcomes of your radiation therapy during the moments of treatment. Focus your mind to visualize the power of the technology going to work with your own disease-fighting mechanism to regain your health and strength.

Plan a visit with friends or family or some other fun, simple activity after the day's treatment.

Talking about the Treatment and the Illness

Great strength can come from talking with others about your reactions to the radiation therapy and the experience of fighting a serious disease. Family, friends, those who have experienced what you are going through, or a counselor can help tremendously by listening to your concerns and responding with empathy.

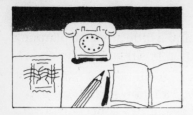

Resources about Radiation Therapy

Booklets

"Radiation Therapy and You: A Guide to Self-Help During Treatment," National Cancer Institute. Bethesda, Maryland 20892. 1985.

This thorough but easy-to-read booklet provides a helpful explanation of what radiation therapy is and how it works. The booklet outlines common side effects of radiation therapy in particular areas of the body receiving treatment and provides suggestions for coping with them. The booklet contains a glossary of frequently used terms relating specifically to radiation therapy.

"Eating Hints: Recipes and Tips for Better Nutrition During Cancer Treatment," NIH Publication No. 84-2079. National Cancer Institute, Bethesda, Maryland 20892.

A spiral-bound booklet that offers easy-to-prepare recipes as well as practical information and advice for eating well during cancer treatment. The booklet is based on patient interviews and lists numerous suggestions to cope with particular problems, including nausea and vomiting, loss of appetite, mouth soreness or dryness, feeling tired, and intestinal upset. "Eating Hints" gives tips for adding protein and calories to meals and suggests options for patients needing soft food or food that is low in fat or fiber.

Main dish, sauce and gravy, and dessert recipes are included to address the particular problems of cancer patients. The recipes are specifically created to be nutritious, easy to make, and tasty for the entire family.

Tapes

"Relaxation and Imagery for the Person with Cancer," by Lynn Brallier, helps persons with cancer to relax, restore their energy, and build a positive base for gaining control of their experience with cancer. The tape helps develop methods and imagery for deep relaxation, which may enhance the effectiveness of medical procedures while supporting the immune system's battle against the cancer cells. This audio tape may be purchased for $10.95 from the Stress/Health Management Center, 621 Maryland Avenue N.E., Washington, D.C. 20002.

CHAPTER SEVEN

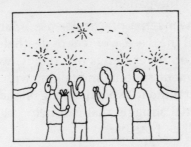

Gathering and Maintaining Emotional Strength and Support

As you use certain disease-fighting mechanisms such as surgery, chemotherapy, and radiation therapy, you can also engage a number of other things in the wellness battle. Whether you consider sharing your feelings with a counselor, talking over events with caring, supportive friends or fellow patients, or making essential changes about how you live your life, you can be aware that these techniques can have a significant impact on your well-being.

Elmo R. Zumwalt III described in an interview for this book how he gathered and maintained emotional strength. He was able to draw successfully on his experiences in youth with serious illnesses, his experiences in Vietnam, and his philosophy of life to support him and his family emotionally as he faced a rare combination of Hodgkin's disease and non-Hodgkin's lymphoma. The treatment that he endured included radiation therapy, chemotherapy, and a painful bone marrow transplant.

"My objective," Zumwalt told me, "was to keep my mind concentrated on the right topics and move forward to make the experience as positive as possible. I decided," he explained, "that the worst thing is not that I should know I might die, but that I might know that and not live my life to the fullest. This is the vital lesson for the person with a terminal illness and for those loved ones who support the patient.

"What this means in a practical sense," Zumwalt continued, "is not to let fear of the disease or fear of death destroy your mind. Focus your mind on other things like family, work, financial arrangements, treatment options, and talking with others in order to cope. Control your mind to avoid dwelling on sadness and depression. It's an internal struggle that can help you get through the experience as well as possible.

"Someone once said," Zumwalt remarked, " 'They who live well die well.' And that's what I concentrated on. I realized I was forever changed by the experience and worked to make it positive. Sure I was afraid. And I am not afraid to be afraid. Fear is a natural feeling and it can be dealt with and faced head on.

"The secret," Zumwalt told me, "is not to dwell on death, but to fight off those thoughts and concentrate on the many things that have to be done that are helpful and make a difference."

Zumwalt reminds us to "keep the mind concentrated on the right topics," because the mind and emotions play a tremendous role in helping the body to gain the full benefits of medical care to combat the invasion of cancer cells.

Talking about It With a Counselor

One crucial decision I made was to use the services of a therapist to help myself deal with and be totally honest about all aspects of the experience. Sharing my feelings with another person helped me to emerge from a sense of unreality and disorientation and come to a clearer understanding of my role in fighting the disease.

Also, getting professional counseling was essential for me because, in addition to cancer threatening my health, other aspects of my life seemed particularly overwhelming. Work responsibilities seemed overly demanding and my personal life was marked by over involvement in too many "good causes," however valuable and enjoyable. Counseling allowed me to begin to get control over those overwhelming circumstances by making changes. These included learning to say no to exciting, but demanding, personal opportunities, beginning the search for new professional opportunities within my company, and learning to cope day-to-day with a life-threatening disease and its treatment.

People who have a loving family member or friend to confide in are fortunate to have such vital support. With or without this support, it is useful to have a professional counselor who is trained to provide another perspective and to be a valuable resource throughout the fight against cancer.

Psychiatrists, psychologists, social workers, psychiatric/mental health nurses, mental health counselors, and pastoral counselors are all trained to help others work through the natural, normal reactions of denial, disorientation, anger, and depression and to help them move toward acceptance, coping, and healing.

A professional counselor also may be able to help you identify and modify ways of reacting to conflicts in day-to-day situations during your treatment and recovery that drain and misdirect energy or keep the body from responding efficiently to the disease or the treatment. The counselor also can provide the support and encouragement that can make it easier to bring about the difficult changes that promote a happier, healthier, longer life.

It is especially useful to find a counselor who understands the disease and is experienced in working with cancer patients. Ask your family doctor, surgeon, radiologist, or medical oncologist for recommendations. Call your local American Cancer Society office, because some local offices have experienced counselors available free of charge for individual or group discussions. Talk with others who have gone through what you are facing to see whom they have worked with and can recommend.

See the resources section at the end of this chapter for information about finding a counselor and learning how to make the experience of therapy as productive as possible.

Using the Cancer Diagnosis as Motivation for Change

Think about the possiblity that a cancer diagnosis can turn out to be the best motivation possible for changing important facets of your life that might not have been all that good for you.

Be prepared to let go of those things, persons, or jobs in your life that have not supported your physical or emotional well-being while moving closer to those individuals and experiences that are supportive of your well-being. Letting go of the unhealthy things in your life can leave time for those persons and activities that you truly cherish. Dropping a number of demanding acquaintances could allow an old, but neglected, friendship to blossom. Changing to a less demanding job, even if it means less prestige or money, could allow more opportunity to grow closer to family members or significant friends. The diagnosis of cancer may provide you the impetus to re-evaluate and come to terms with the expectations that you and others have imposed on your life, while offering you the opportunity to redirect your interest and energy.

If you think you need one, opt for a change—to give to yourself as well as to others in your life. With or without support from your spouse, friends, family, or boss, you may need to be prepared to let go of or begin to change unhealthy relationships in your life. Start seeing those choices you overlooked before. Unlock yourself as much as possible from unhappy and unhealthy situations. Explore the possibility of taking a temporary leave of absence from your job. Talk with a significant other about the major or minor things you need to change in order to stay healthy and happy.

Realize that your well-being may mean making some changes and that you can begin preparing yourself immediately to work toward them. As you stabilize your emotional condition and begin your healing process, be willing to give yourself permission to change—whether it's your job responsibilities, your spouse, your lifestyle, or your attitudes. Be prepared to confront a demanding or insensitive spouse or parent. Be willing to begin thinking about the implications of more drastic changes such as letting go of an unhealthy relationship or beginning the search for a new job. Ask others for their support as you make these changes.

Taking Care of Yourself

Establish a goal to take care of your own physical and emotional needs. Taking care of yourself can include setting aside time each day and evening to renew yourself and to build up your energy supply through meditation or relaxation response. It can mean doing something that you really want to do—even something small—for someone else or for yourself. It can also include making specific decisions or establishing definite limits for how much you can be involved in.

Helping others—whether through the family, community, religious organizations, schools, or other voluntary groups—can be invigorating and health-giving. Yet chronic over-involvement in even worthwhile activities can be detrimental and energy-sapping.

This is not to suggest that over-involvement in activities causes cancer! It is a reminder that all of us—and especially those of us recovering from cancer—need to take care of our own physical and emotional needs for restoration and renewal. We need to keep our life in a healthy balance and actively listen to the messages our body sends us. This attention can ensure that we do not sacrifice our own well-being by overdoing in any one aspect of our lives, whether it is in our work in or out of the home, serving our family needs, or volunteering in community or social service groups.

Asking Others for Help

Be willing to ask family, friends, health professionals, volunteer agency personnel, and others for their help. Determine what you need or want and ask for help to make it happen. Try to make this difficult time as easy for yourself as possible—whether it is by having someone accompany you to the hospital or doctor's office, having overnight company when you feel ill, or *not* having someone come to visit when company—even loving, well-intentioned guests—would be detrimental to your well-being.

Maintaining Normalcy in Your Life

Try to maintain some sense of normalcy in your schedule by continuing to do the things you enjoy doing. For example, if you love writing post cards during your vacation trips, consider sending post cards from your hospital stay. If you enjoy writing, start a journal about your experiences. If you're an amateur photographer, create an album of pictures of your doctors and nurses and their waiting rooms.

I appreciated maintaining most of my work responsibilities both in the hospital and throughout the year-long recovery because they provided me with a certain regular schedule, a sense of fulfillment in an important part of my life, and a sense of control over events.

My staff and I worked diligently and planned carefully through my hospitalization and recovery periods to complete department projects on schedule. This required unusual flexiblity—such as having a delivery service bring the printer's bluelines to my hospital room for review and handling a lot of meetings and decisions by telephone rather than in person. But because my staff and I wanted to make it work, we did.

I found my ongoing work responsiblities to be a welcome change of pace during tough times. Our department work that year may have turned out better than ever—one of our major projects was honored with a first prize award by a business communicators association.

Talking about It with Supportive Individuals

Talk with others who are going through what you're going through or who have faced a similarly serious illness. This can give you the sense that you're not alone in what you're feeling and how you're coping with the threat of a serious disease.

In many cities, hospital social service departments, the American Cancer Society, and Make Today Count provide support groups led by trained counselors knowledgeable about cancer. These groups are usually free of charge and can provide important, valuable help and support for many patients.

I gained great strength from participating in a breast cancer support group sponsored by a local unit of the American Cancer Society. The day I returned home from the hospital after my first mastectomy, a social worker called to ask how I was doing, tell me about the support group meetings, and ask if I would like a volunteer who had gone through a similar experience of fighting breast cancer to stop by my home for a visit.

Even though my visit with the Reach to Recovery volunteer lasted only an hour or so, meeting and talking with her was, like participating in a support group, an important stage in my recovery. The volunteer not only brought me items to use for physical therapy and showed me how to use them, but she also gave me an opportunity to ask questions about specific concerns I had regarding the days, weeks, and months ahead.

The breast cancer support group meetings offered another opportunity to talk on a regular, ongoing basis about the experience of fighting cancer and to learn how others were facing the same problems and concerns that I had.

My support group varied in size from meeting to meeting, but usually had between five and fifteen participants, with two social workers acting as group leaders. Even though the support group was originally planned to meet weekly for two months, the members decided it was important for us to keep in touch on a monthly basis for as long as we felt the need.

In the hour-and-a-half- to two-hour meetings, we were able to talk about our problems, fears, questions, and difficulties and ask for help and support from others. Sometimes group members needed a referral to a plastic surgeon, oncologist, psychiatrist, or other medical specialist. Other times one of us needed to hear how other members were dealing with sexual or other concerns because of the mastectomy.

Sometimes we talked about our fears of the cancer recurring and shared how we coped with this overriding concern. Many times we gave each other our ways for living healthier lives. We shared information about useful workshops, seminars, articles, or books and presented new information from our doctors that would be of help to someone else.

Contact your local American Cancer Society office or one of the many other agencies that provide support group meetings to patients and their families.

Many organizations also maintain a list of persons who have fought or are fighting the same cancer you are facing who will "buddy-up" with you in person or by phone to give support and to share their experiences and insights. Contact the Cancer Information Service toll-free line, 1-800-4-CANCER, or see the resources section at the end of this chapter for information about support groups and telephone contact lines.

Being Ready for Miracles

Rely on your own power of prayer or on the power of prayers from friends, family, or persons in religious organizations. It can be a tremendous support to know that the force of others' faith and hope are being channeled for your recovery.

My spirit was boosted tremendously by knowing that family, friends, and even health professionals were caring and concerned enough to request prayers for my health from their church congregations, prayer groups, school classmates, and religious communities. I also felt deeply touched and connected in a special way when the family's matriarch, in poor health herself, sent me her health-giving holy water collected years earlier from a shrine in Lourdes.

Be prepared to have new friends that you can lean on enter your life. Be open for the miracle of their friendship to present itself at difficult times. At the same time, don't be surprised if some friends fall away from you when they learn you have cancer. You'll never know why—whether it's their inability to deal with illness or the threat of death or that they just don't know what to say or how to relate to someone with a serious illness.

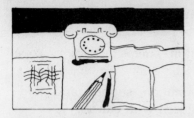

Resources for Gathering and Maintaining Emotional Strength and Support

Opportunities for Support

Many local, regional, and national agencies offer opportunities for support in addition to their other services and programs. A number of the well-known ones follow. For more information about these agencies, their services, and their addresses and telephone numbers, see the resources section for Chapter One, Immediate Mobilization. Contact the social service department of your hospital, your local American Cancer Society office, or the Cancer Information Service—1-800-4-CANCER—for comprehensive information about opportunities for support, hot lines, or other service groups to contact in your area.

CanSurmount or Can Support—a one-on-one visitor program of the American Cancer Society that provides trained volunteers (many are also former cancer patients) to visit with other cancer patients, their families, health professionals, and the public. The volunteers provide emotional support and useful information. The CanSurmount program also provides educational programs and professional in-service workshops for health professionals.

ENCORE—a discussion and exercise program of the Y.W.C.A. for women who have had breast cancer surgery.

Reach to Recovery—A one-on-one visitor program of The American Cancer Society for women with breast cancer.

The Lost Chord/Laryngectomy Patient Rehabilitation Program of the American Cancer Society.

The **Ostomy Rehabilitation Program of The American Cancer Society.**

The **United Ostomy Association**—helps ostomates cope with everyday experiences.

Candlelighters—provides information, support and guidance for parents and families of children with cancer.

The **Leukemia Society of America**—has local chapters that may offer support groups for patients and their families.

Make Today Count—has group meetings and a telephone contact support system for patients and their families who are facing life-threatening illness.

The **United Cancer Council**—has local affiliates that offer patient and family support groups.

Community Telephone Lines for Contact and Support

Many communities have an agency that offers a telephone line to provide assistance and support to cancer patients and their families. Contact your local Cancer Information Service for information about the existence of a cancer "Hot Line" or "Contact Line" in your city, county, or state.

A few of the many cancer hot lines are described below:

ARKANSAS

Little Rock

501-660-3900

Toll Free: 1-800-632-4614 (within Arkansas)

Hours: 8 A.M. to 4:30 P.M. (Central Standard), Monday through Friday

Services: Former cancer patients or their family members offer advice, emotional support, and their own experience. Callers are matched with the patient-volunteers for similar disease, age, and sex.

Additional Services: A social worker is available to callers, also.

Additional Information: Printed information may be requested.

FLORIDA

Broward and Dade Counties

305-721-7600

Hours: 9 A.M.-3:30 P.M., Monday through Friday. (Calls are forwarded on weekends to volunteers' homes.)

Services: Former cancer patients or their families offer a listening ear, emotional support, information, and advice. Patients are matched with a "buddy"—survivors of similar age, sex, medications, and disease. The Hot Line provides referral suggestions for such services as home care agencies, medical services, counseling, transportation assistance, and financial help.

Additional Information: Monthly newsletter.

MISSOURI

Kansas City

816-932-8453

Hours: 9 A.M. to 5 P.M. (Central Standard), Monday through Friday

Services: Former cancer patients or their family members offer advice, emotional support, and the value of their own experiences. Callers are matched with the patient-volunteers for similar disease, age, and sex.

Other Information: Two books by Richard and Annette Bloch, *Fighting Cancer* ($4.00) and *Cancer, There's Hope* ($3.00), and a guided imagery relaxation tape for stress and pain management ($5.00) are available for purchase or loan. These materials are available free to libraries and clergy on request.

OHIO

Cincinnati

CancerShare

513-221-3030

Hours: 9 A.M. to 3:00 P.M. (Eastern Standard), Monday through Friday. (At other times, callers can leave a message on the answering machine.)

Services: Trained voluteers who have had a personal experience with cancer talk with patients and/or their family members to answer non-medical questions, offer support, and help meet caller's needs. Callers are matched to volunteers by type of cancer, treatment, age, and specific needs callers identify.

Additional Information: CancerShare has books available for loan by written or phone request.

Cleveland

216-292-8222

Hours: 9 A.M. to 5 P.M. (Eastern Standard), Monday through Friday

Services: Former cancer patients or their family members offer positive, emotional support as well as the value of their experience. Callers are matched with the former patient-volunteers for similar disease, age, and sex.

OKLAHOMA

Oklahoma City
The Cancer Connection

405-949-3000

Hours: 8:00 A.M. to 4:30 P.M. (Central Standard), Monday through Friday. (At other times, callers can leave a message on the answering machine.)

Services: Trained volunteers who have had a personal experience with cancer talk with patients and/or their family members through a telephone support network. Callers are matched with volunteers for similar disease, age, sex, and treatment.

PENNSYLVANIA

Pittsburgh
The Cancer Guidance Institute

412-782-4023

Hours: Calls are answered twenty-four hours a day.

Services: Cancer patients offer advice, emotional support, and their own experience. The trained patient-volunteers provide compassion as well as information on community services and resources.

Additional Information: Quarterly newsletter, *Living with Cancer* by Lynn Gray, is sent free on request. The relaxation tape, "Mind Over Cancer" ($11) can be ordered.

WASHINGTON

Seattle
Cancer LifeLine

206-447-4542

Hours: Twenty-four hours a day, seven days a week

Services: Well trained volunteers provide supportive counseling, information, and community resources to cancer patients, their families, and friends. They help callers clarify problems and concerns, identify possible solutions, locate information and community resources, and find ways to communicate more effectively with family, friends, and health professionals.

Additional Information: Cancer Lifeline also provides programs for public education and family conferences as well as workplace seminars and consultations.

Books

The Road Back to Health: Coping With The Emotional Side of Cancer,
Neil A. Fiore, Bantam Books, 1986.

> *The Road Back to Health,* a valuable book by a psychologist who is also a cancer patient, provides thoughtful, practical advice for coping with the many demands of cancer. Chapter

titles include "Coping With the Diagnosis," "The Power of Your Beliefs," "Becoming an Active Patient," "You and Your Doctor," "Making Decisions About Your Cancer Therapy," "Communicating with Family and Friends," "Communication Skills," "Coping with Depression and Helplessness," "Managing the Stress of Cancer," and "Coping with Terminal Illness." Appendixes provide an exercise for dealing with the diagnosis, information about getting treatment and support, a stress log, a Patient's Bill of Rights, and documents about care at the end of life.

Anatomy of an Illness, Norman Cousins, Norton, 1979.

Anatomy of an Illness describes how Norman Cousins, facing the pain and uncertainty of a life-threatening illness, developed a partnership with his doctor to exploit the power of his mind, his strong will to live, ascorbic acid therapy, and lots of laughter from "Candid Camera" television shows and Marx brothers movies to turn around and then stop the course of his disease.

Cousins examines the vital role that the mind plays in conquering disease, the importance of trust between patients and their doctors and the trust patients have in the medications their doctors prescribe. His personal and inspiring story has helped many people suffering from serious illnesses, while pointedly relating how mysterious, still, is the relationship among mind, body, and emotion.

Cousins reviews the development of the holistic health movement and shares with the reader the responses of doctors and patients or their families who welcome his ideas and support the methods he used to bring about his inspiring success.

My Father, My Son, Admiral Elmo Zumwalt, Jr., Lieutenant Elmo Zumwalt III with John Pekkanen, Macmillian, New York, 1986.

An inspiring story of the experiences of the Admiral, son Elmo, grandson Russell, and other family members and their courage in adversity. Cancer patients can learn powerful coping skills from the Zumwalt family and Elmo's experiences fighting a rare combination of cancers.

Transition and Transformation: Successfully Managing Stress, Lynn Brallier, National Nursing Review, Los Altos, California, 1982.

Successfully Managing Stress examines the potential for stress that comes from every aspect of living—home life, work life, friends, our bodies and minds, our emotions, our self-concept, our personality, and our spiritual beliefs and values. Numerous self-assessment tests and checklists, along with follow-up explanations, allow readers to identify and analyze potential problems with managing their stress.

The book is packed with practical how to techniques to manage stress through exercise, proper nutrition, various meditation procedures, biofeedback techniques, imagery, time management, accommodation to stress, assertiveness styles, coping mechanisms, goal setting, and decision making. One section presents creative, but practical, ways to deal with stressful emotions or troubles such as fear, anger, guilt, anxiety, depression, loneliness, insomnia, perfectionism, and substance addiction.

Stress Without Distress, Hans Selye, Harper & Row, New York, 1974.

Stress Without Distress provides a readable explanation, based on this research scientist's findings, of what stress and distress are and how they differ in their impact on the body. Selye describes his "General Adaptation Syndrome" and illustrates how the body typically reacts to stress—the alarm stage, followed by the body's action of resistance, followed by its response of exhaustion. Selye believes that the body contains only a finite amount of adaptation energy in order to respond to stress throughout life. Each person's unique store of adaptation energy affects the person's ability to stay alive and healthy.

Selye offers suggestions for ways of maximizing life-long satisfaction while minimizing loss of adaptation energy. His suggestions require that readers consider their long- and short-term goals in life, and the basic philosophy on which their life is based. He offers his own specific suggestions for ways to achieve a full, satisfying life.

When Talk is Not Cheap or How to Find the Right Therapist When You Don't Know How to Begin, Mandy Aftel, M.A., M.F.C.C., and Robin Tolmach Lakoff, Ph.D., Warner Books, New York, 1985.

This book acquaints readers with the many important issues involved in making the experience of psychotherapy as meaningful as possible. These issues include how to determine if psychotherapy would be helpful, how to locate a therapist who would be best, how to work with and relate to the therapist, and how to recognize if, or when, the experience is not productive. The authors provide numerous checklists and exercises to aid the reader in making decisions about starting or stopping therapy, selecting a therapist, determining therapy goals, evaluating the relationship with the therapist, and identifying progress made from therapy.

The authors include follow-up readings on most topics as well as a glossary of basic terms.

Booklets

"Taking Time—Support for People With Cancer and the People Who Care About Them," U.S. Department of Health and Human Services, National Institutes of Health, Publication No. 83-2059.

This booklet examines feelings and emotional problems involved in facing cancer and describes how others have learned to cope. The materials offer suggestions for sharing feelings, dealing with friends, and solving problems within the family. The booklet provides ideas about where and how to find emotional and practical assistance.

Periodicals

Advances, the quarterly journal of the Institute for the Advancement of Health. *Advances,* oriented to health professionals and interested members of the general public, explores such issues as how the mind and body interact to affect health and disease. Articles include a brief summary of main points. The publication also includes a calendar of upcoming workshops or conferences and a short description of studies in progress.

CHAPTER EIGHT

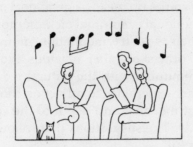

Keeping Your Spirits Up

In the Broadway play, "The Search for Signs of Intelligent Life in the Universe," written by Jane Wagner and starring Lily Tomlin, Trudy the bag woman says, "If evolution were worth its salt, by now it should have evolved something better than 'survival of the fittest'; a better idea would be 'survival of the wittiest.' At least that way, the creatures that *didn't* survive could've died *laughing*."

Something magical happens to our bodies, minds, and spirits when we can laugh and be tickled or amused. Scientists have shown that laughter triggers the brain to release certain chemicals in the body—endorphins—that can block pain and give a sense of well-being. And those of us who aren't scientists have experienced the feelings of pleasure and relief of tension that come from sharing a good laugh.

Getting well and staying well can be enhanced, and is certainly more fun, when laughter is part of the healing prescription. The road back to good health can encompass so many experiences, including surgery, a modification in diet, radiation therapy, physical therapy, chemotherapy, psychotherapy, and a range of vital "spiritual" resources and techniques. Laughter is definitely one of these vital resources for healing power.

Keeping your spirits up means a great deal more than laughter, though. An emotional or spiritual pick-me-up can come from a variety of forces such as poetry, meditation, motivational or inspirational readings, prayer or other religious experiences, artistic expression, or communing with the natural world. Each person can search his or her experience to reflect on those special things that add a sense of meaning and depth to the spirit and help to heal the ailing body. The suggestions that follow are some ideas you may find helpful.

Setting Aside Time to Keep Things Light

Go out to see a funny, fanciful, or heart-warming movie, or borrow one to play at home if you have a video cassette recorder. Four days after my cancer diagnosis, while I was very much caught up in the flurry of getting second opinions, bone and liver scans, and pulling together all the resources I could, I went with family and friends to see a film with lots of whimsy, caring, and laughs. It helped all of us put aside our problems for an hour or two and return to them later feeling refreshed and inspired.

Watch funny TV shows or tape them to see later to add some chuckles to your life.

Borrow comedy records or audio tapes from friends or the public library. Use a portable tape player and earphones to listen to comedy tapes during waits in doctors' offices or in the hospital. I found the best way to stir myself out of bed after chemotherapy treatments was to listen to a favorite comedian on tape. Getting to know the jokes after several hearings only seemed to add to the enjoyment.

Read the comic pages in the newspaper daily. Save your favorites in an envelope to keep with you. Pull out the comic strips to read whenever your spirits need a quick boost—in doctors' waiting rooms, waiting for the bus or train to go to the doctors; or to use on those days before chemotherapy or radiation therapy appointments.

When one of my doctors asked to see my cartoon collection, I decided to publish the contents for friends as my *Christmas Cheer* holiday gift. The comic strip creators and syndicates cooperated by giving me permission to republish their copyrighted material to share with friends. All of this was accomplished in the spirit of "getting more humor into our lives."

Start a humor journal in which you jot down daily funny things you see, hear, or read. Keeping a humor journal helps put more humor into each day by providing the motivation for looking for humor—and seeing it—in all situations and at all times.

Filling the Spirit with Good Things

Create a Health and Happiness Shelf at home, in the hospital, or in some other private space where you keep your own spirit boosters—your favorite books of poetry or motivation, your humor books, the prayers or meditations that speak to you, your favorite greeting cards, and other items that amuse and delight. Know that you can come to this shelf at any time to select from a variety of special, familiar mementos that will give you help and strength. Keep adding to the shelf and enlarging its capacity to respond to the needs of your spirit.

My best friend gave me a loving cup trophy to mark my accomplishments in a year of trials. That trophy became the centerpiece of my Health and Happiness Shelf.

Get re-involved in some activity that gave you great joy, inspiration, and spiritual uplift at some time in your life. Renew a hobby from healthy days. If you got great joy and satisfaction from singing in the church choir as a teenager or college student, try joining a group that can help you re-experience that joy and inner pleasure now.

Keep a personal journal to record your thoughts and feelings. The turmoil of the spirit that accompanies a serious illness is natural. Keeping a record of your feelings helps you recognize the change and growth within you that naturally occurs from such turmoil.

Attach yourself to things in nature that you love or appreciate which have a particular natural cycle that you can follow and use as your own natural calendar. For example, if you begin your recovery in the spring and you know that certain spring flowers set out in April will grow, bloom, and enlarge while continuing to rebloom, you can mark your own progress with the cycle of the flowers.

Plan something major and fun for yourself when you have recovered. This gives you something special and definite for which you can plan and look ahead.

When I was about 25 percent finished with my chemotherapy treatments, I decided a friend and I would take a long vacation in Italy and France the spring following my recovery. This decision meant that I had eight or nine months to clip articles, write for maps and brochures, study Italian, and tell people about the trip we were planning.

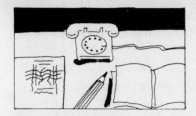

Resources for Keeping Your Spirits Up

Materials Available for Loan

Laughter Therapy
Allen Funt Productions
P.O. Box 827
Monterey, CA 93940
408-625-3788

Warning! Laughter may be hazardous to your illness. Spend three hours chuckling at antics from TV's classic comedy series *Candid Camera*. A "Best of Candid Camera" videotape may be borrowed free of charge. Written requests are preferred, but telephone orders are accepted.

Workshops

"The Power of Laughter and Play"—a two-and-a-half day conference—examines the powerful force that laughter and play can be for patients who are seriously ill or in pain. Call or write for information about locations and dates to The Institute for the Advancement of Human Behavior, 4370 Alpine Road, Suite 108, Portola Valley, California 94025, 415-851-8411.

Conference presentations are available on a twelve-audio tape set for $98. What follows is a partial list of titles: *Stress Management and Humor* (2 tapes) by Steve Allen, Jr., M.D., LPC15, $16.95; *Uses of Humor: How to Be Systematically Outrageous* by Richard Bandler LP107, $9.95; *Humor and Health: The Physiology and Emotional Effects of Laugher* by Alison Crane, B.S.N., R.N., LP306, $9.95; *The Clinical Use of Humor: Putting the Healing Force of Humor into Practice* (2 tapes) by Alison Crane, B.S.N., R.N., LP308, $16.95; *The Magic of Humor: A Ho-Ho-Holistic View* by Joel

Goodman, Ed.D., LP108, $9.95; *Humor & Death: You've Got to be Kidding* (2 tapes) by Allen Klein, M.A., LPC9, $16.95; *Growing Young: The Functions of Laughter and Play,* by Ashley Montagu, Ph.D., LP110, $9.95; *Humor as a Therapeutic Intervention* by Raymond Moody, M.D., LP114, $9.95; *Paradox, Humor and Healing* by Gerald W. Piaget, Ph.D., LP100, $9.95; and *Functions of Humor in the Health Professions* (2 tapes) by Vera M. Robinson, R.N., Ed.D., LPC13, $16.95. For a complete list contact the Institute.

"The Positive Power of Humor and Creativity"—a two-and-a-half day workshop that brings together more than a dozen faculty in a country resort location of the Adirondack Mountains to work and play with a light look at the serious subject of humor and creativity. The conference provides opportunities to learn and practice ways of tapping into your own sense of humor and creativity and to recognize ways of integrating humor and creativity into your life, work, and recovery to health. For more information on this conference and other programs throughout the United States and abroad, contact Dr. Joel Goodman, Director, The Humor Project, 110 Spring Street, Saratoga Springs, New York 12866; 518-587-8770.

"The Healing Power of Humor"—which demonstrates the therapeutic benefits of humor, and "Humor and Death: You've Got to Be Kidding," which shows the outstanding coping and communicating qualities of humor, are one-day workshops offered by Allen Klein/The Whole Mirth Catalog, 1034 Page Street, San Francisco, California 94117; 415-431-1913.

Adult Camps

Camp Bluebird
St. Vincent Hospital
2701 Ninth Court South
Birmingham, Alabama 35201
205-939-7000

A three-day adult camp held in April and October for those eighteen and older in the countryside near Birmingham, Alabama, for patients in all stages of fighting cancer to develop independent living skills and participate in programs on wellness, pain control, relaxation and visual imagery. In addition, the camp provides all the camping experiences you knew as a kid—boating, horseback riding, crafts, and campfires. Special diets and medical staff are available. Camp counselors are doctors, nurses, social workers, hospice nurses, and pastoral care counselors who volunteer their time.

Adult and Youth Camps

Colorado Outward Bound School
945 Pennsylvania Street
Denver, Colorado 80302
303-837-0880
Contact: Director, Health Services Program

Cancer patients, their families and friends, and health professionals can participate in three-day Outward Bound courses with activities specifically geared toward those whose lives are touched by cancer. Outward Bound uses the wilderness and the group experience as a means for persons to learn about themselves. Each course is tailored to individuals enrolled in the course. For persons twelve years of age and older. Cost $160.

Children's Camps

Summer camp can be just what the doctor ordered whether for the child with cancer or for siblings or parents of children with cancer. Contact your physician or hospital social worker, the Cancer Information Service, or your local American Cancer Society office for camp names and contacts.

Periodicals

Laughing Matters. Four issues per year published by The Humor Project, 110 Spring Street, Saratoga Springs, New York 12866. $15 per year. Back issues available at $25 for two years, $33 for three years, or $40 for four years.

Editor Joel Goodman, director of The Humor Project, presents practical, real life techniques for getting more humor in life and work. Issues feature an interview with a comedy great, such as Steve Allen, Dom DeLuise, Allen Funt, Gene Perret, Charles Schulz, or Norman Cousins. In addition, all issues include fun-filled information such as "Discover the Elf in Yourself," "Grin and Share It," "The Laughter Prescription,"

"Readers' Di-Jest," "How to Develop Your Own Sense of Humor—Swiftly," "Fun-Liners Jest for You," and many more.

Catalogs

The Whole Mirth Catalog, 1034 Page Street, San Francisco, California 94117. Send $1.50 to cover postage and handling. This newspaper-format catalog offers every playful and light-hearted product imaginable—from comic rubber stamps and funny nose masks to designer trash bags and comedy tapes. One section of *The Whole Mirth Catalog* also presents books, newsletters, directories, and other catalogs oriented to jokes, humor, or laughter for children and adults.

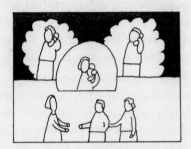

CHAPTER NINE

Communicating with Your Family and Friends

It is essential that persons with cancer be able to admit their illness and discuss the ramifications of it with their spouses, family, or other important persons in their lives. This is not only the case for persons with cancer, of course, but for those with other chronic diseases or addictions as well. The spouse, family, and other loved ones need to be involved in communication and decision making because their lives are so deeply affected by the patient's health and well-being.

When You Need to Be Encouraged to Talk

Because issues of health affect the spouse or other loved ones so completely, it is essential that the patient be willing and able to talk about the short- and long-term impact this illness may have. Together they can mobilize and respond to the disease and openly share their feelings with each other about their experiences.

Sometimes the spouse or other loved one needs to encourage or even push the patient to discuss these issues. Facing a cancer diagnosis is such a painful and stressful experience that it can make communication difficult and stressful. For the spouse or loved ones to be shut out from the patient's feelings deprives them of their right and responsiblity to offer comfort and empathy to the patient or advice and perspective on the patient's decisions. For the person with cancer to believe that the illness is just his or her problem and no one else's is taking too narrow a view of life.

This lesson was clarified for me when a long-time friend and his wife discussed how they had to work through the barriers of communicating about her chronic disease, diabetes. While they were dating, she resisted any attempt he made to discuss her diabetes. She believed that the diabetes was her problem and something she had no need or reason to discuss with him. She could continue to handle her diabetes successfully on her own. If he loved her and enjoyed being with her, that was all that mattered.

My friend wanted to be included in all dimensions of her life and well-being, including the important part of her life relating to her diabetes. He needed to talk with her about his frustrations and feelings of rejection and about feeling excluded from the valuable opportunities to be compassionate and supportive of her experiences with diabetes.

After several discussions, she realized that sharing information with him about her illness was not putting a burden on him or making her less attractive to him, but was allowing him to be involved more fully and intimately in her life.

Dealing with the Anger of Others

Some spouses or other loved ones may react with anger at any effort of the patient to discuss the illness or proposed treatment. A member of my support group recounted her experience with her husband when she informed him that she needed to have a biopsy. He responded with anger, implied that her illness was ruining their social life, and sulked about the amount of time she would need to recuperate.

This angry response, based in his insecurity, feelings of hopelessness, and fear of losing a valuable part of his life, created a confused, hopeless state for the patient and only further encouraged her to feel victimized and to hide her thoughts and feelings from her spouse. As painful and frightening as it was for her, she needed to try to address her husband's barrier of anger with him and turn it into something creative and worthwhile if possible. In this way they could have more open, complete discussions about his fears of being abandoned and his feelings about and responsibility for helping her fight this disease.

Talking about Your Feelings

The common reaction that many patients face is that friends and family members initially have a hard time letting the patient talk honestly about fears and concerns. Quite a few family members and friends mistakenly believe, at least at first, that it is their responsibility to cheer up and keep the patient happy. They may consequently tend to discourage the patient from talking seriously about the fears and feelings that come from managing a serious disease.

While being optimistic about recovery is very important, a false cheerfulness from family and friends can be very discouraging and depressing. Patients secretly wonder how these cheerful people must really feel when they dismiss a patient's concerns with such statements as "Let's think happy thoughts" or, "Don't be silly. Of course, you'll be fine."

I think most patients face this experience at some time during their illness—whether from family or well-meaning friends. Whenever I would begin to talk about my apprehensions about the surgery, chemotherapy, recurrence, or follow-up examinations, my family would interrupt me with a loving, but firm, "Now, don't talk like that. That's silly. You're going to be just fine!"

While loved ones use this approach in an effort to make the patient feel better, it is difficult to deal with because this response does not allow any opportunity to talk about poignant fears and concerns that need to be discussed.

It is essential to talk with these loved ones honestly to make them aware of just how important it is to discuss your fears and concerns openly with them. If you do not let them know that their bouncy, "all will be well" style is bothersome and depressing, they will most likely continue that approach, believing all the while that this constant dose of optimism is in your best interest.

I was fortunate to be able to talk through my fears about the disease and the treatment with a friend and a counselor. They let me describe my fears. They emphathized with me and expressed their frustration that the reality of cancer is that no one, for sure, knows whether you'll get well and stay well.

They listened to my fears and agreed with me that fighting cancer is a scary thing. They assured me that it is a normal, human reaction to be scared. At the same time, they reminded me that I was doing absolutely everything that modern medicine knows how to do to fight cancer, as well as some alternative measures in the form of relaxation, stress management, and humor that might be useful, too. They encouraged me to talk with members of my support group to see how they dealt with their fears and apprehensions.

Loved ones do a great service when they allow and encourage patients to discuss openly and honestly their range of feelings and fears. Sometimes these feelings may be gloomy or fearful; other times they may be optimistic and cheery. The important thing is that patients feel free to talk about their feelings and know that their loved ones will listen with care.

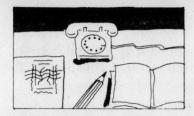

Resources for Communicating with Your Family and Friends

Books

The Healing Family: The Simonton Approach for Families Facing Illness, Stephanie Matthews-Simonton and Robert Shook. Bantam, 1984.

The Healing Family provides practical suggestions to assist the patient, his or her family, or other loved ones communicate their feelings in open and healthy ways and to be helpful and mutually supportive.

Ms. Simonton gives ways the family can mobilize itself both individually and as a team. She suggests ways for the family to gather medical information and maintain hope while adapting to the diagnosis of cancer and supporting the patient in his or her need to fight the illness and make dramatic lifestyle changes.

Ms. Simonton offers practical reminders for overcoming the fear associated with the cancer diagnosis and suggests helpful ways to assist the patient to recognize and deal with his or her feelings of fear or depression. She gives suggestions to assist patients and their families who face cancer recurrence or death.

Ms. Simonton reminds us of the positive outcomes possible from cancer—a willingness to express feelings, a heightened appreciation of life, a discovery of self-worth and an interest in taking better care of the body through closer attention to habits of sleep, nutrition and exercise.

The Road Back to Health: Coping With The Emotional Side of Cancer,
Neil A. Fiore, Bantam Books, 1986.

Fiore, a psychologist and cancer patient, offers valuable advice for patients facing difficulties communicating with family and friends.

Chapter Six, "Communicating With Family and Friends," includes sections such as "Coping With the Reactions of Others," "Feeling Isolated," "Changes in Relationships," "Changes in Family Roles" and "Barriers to Communication." Chapter Seven, "Communication Skills," includes useful discussions such as "Why Share Your Feelings?" "Controlling Your Thoughts," "Speaking the Unspeakable" and "Three Essential Skills."

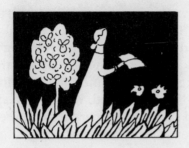

CHAPTER TEN

Working Toward Quality Living

Fighting cancer and staying cancer-free is a lifelong process. Because cancer is a chronic disease, it demands the greatest vigilance and attention, both during the recovery period and during times of remission.

Having cancer means living the rest of your life with the uncertainty of possible recurrence. It is a painful realization, but an essential one, if we are going to be alert to the fight and work toward achieving peace and a high quality life even after a diagnosis of cancer.

We have to be always on the alert in the fight against cancer. This can be a difficult message to accept, but it is not intended to paralyze the recovering patient. Instead, it is intended to make clear that the disease is one whose origin and progress are not completely known or understood. Because of this, it is in the patient's best interest to accept every opportunity and every precious moment of life as a special gift to be used and enjoyed.

Staying Aware of Developments in the Fight with Cancer

Several things are vital in our efforts to live with the uncertainty of cancer recurrence. These include going for regular check-ups with our physicians and being alert to any warning signs our bodies send. In addition, keeping informed about the latest in cancer control may aid our acceptance of cancer and provide support for the constant vigilance that is required. When we keep current, we can be more active and savvy consumers of health services during the fight against cancer or its recurrence.

A source of current information is *Cope*, a magazine for cancer patients, their families, and health professionals. The magazine was started to make sure patients and families touched by cancer have access to the latest news about the disease. It is written in a clear, nontechnical style and highlights current thinking about treatments and ways of coping with the disease. See the resources section at the end of this chapter for subscription information.

If you find that you are not interested in researching or reading this kind of information, or you are not able to, consider asking one of your "readers," a support person described in Chapter One, to assist you with this reading.

As I stay aware of developments in the fight against cancer, I find it useful to gain insight from counselors who help me look from a fresh perspective at my lifestyle and patterns and ways of responding to challenges and conflicts. These counselors help me to see and explore new styles and patterns that are more beneficial to my well-being than the well-established ones I was used to.

This effort to change involves a number of things such as paying attention to having medical check-ups on schedule, following sound nutritional guidelines, watching that alcohol is consumed in moderation, paying careful attention to managing stress through biofeedback, using meditation, and making time for exercise regularly. All of these things make me feel that I am doing as much as possible to stay healthy and to aid my immune system in any battles with cancer cells.

Some experts in the field believe that it is a very healthy response to put the experience of cancer behind you and move on with your life. One cannot or need not be a cancer "patient" forever.

Finding Home Health Care Services

Some cancer patients or their families may find that certain home health care services are especially helpful at certain times during the illness. Home health care can include everything from personal and homemaking assistance to registered nursing service, licensed practical nursing assistance, nurses' aides, therapists (physical, occupational rehabilitation, speech), and specialized home health care assistance, such as to administer chemotherapy treatments.

In order to find the most appropriate home health care for your needs, contact your hospital social services department or the hospital discharge planning personnel to elicit their recommendations. Ask your doctor or contact your local office of the American Cancer Society, which may be able to offer recommendations or direct you to county or city social service agencies. See the resources section at the end of this chapter for more information about home health care service options.

Recognizing Our Mortality to Enhance Quality Living

Growth and change can come from a number of different events or crises that confront us throughout our lives. Loss of a loved one or the struggle to face one's own death can provide dramatic opportunities to recognize and give thanks for one's existence.

It is by accepting our mortality that we can come to appreciate the essential pleasures and wonder of our life. The fact that our life does end gives meaning and worth to the time we have—time that is limited, special, and not able to be repeated. Just like the message on the button, "Enjoy Life. This is *Not* a Dress Rehearsal," the acceptance of our mortality can be an opportunity to experience life fully and cherish the precious moments we have. Accepting our mortality offers us reason to concentrate on the present moments we have to enjoy, rather than spending major portions of our life looking back or living for the future.

Coming face-to-face with our mortality or coping with the death of a loved one is not an easy task. It is painful and frightening. It is something we do not really know how to do. It requires struggle, growth, and change. One of the things that acceptance of our mortality offers us is the opportunity to live a life that is fuller and richer and more concentrated in the present moment.

Using Hospice Programs to Help Face Death

Coping with our mortality is a frightening experience. Sometimes the fear and apprehension comes from the question of what it will be like for us at the end. We fear what the process of death will be like. We wonder if it will be full of pain, isolation, and loss of dignity. It is natural to have a fear of dying—maybe even dying alone—in strange surroundings with the latest medical equipment and devices impinging into the hallowed area where we want our caring loved ones to be.

While hospitals and nursing homes may offer patients the specialized services and advanced medical technology they require to fight the disease or its symptoms and stave off death, some cancer patients may find that the support from a hospice program can be a fulfillment of their particular preference for their final days.

Hospice programs offer terminally ill patients and their families the opportunity for appropriate medical care and attention to the patient who remains more at peace in the familiar, comforting surroundings of the home. In some cases, when the patient's home setting is not appropriate, the terminally ill patient can be served at a local hospice facility. The quality caring that hospice patients receive—whether at home or in the hospice environment—is largely provided by trained volunteers and family members.

The hospice team is actively involved with the family and is on call around-the-clock to offer care and comfort to the terminally ill patient. The hospice team comprises a hospice physician, hospice nurse, social worker, chaplain, aides, volunteers, and others to provide a variety of medical care as well as emotional support.

The medical care includes attending to the patient's needs for such things as pain control medication and relief from unwanted symptoms. The emotional support includes attending to the psychological and spiritual needs of the patient and family as they confront death. These services are provided outside of an "acute care" environment in the familiar, comfortable surroundings of the patient's home or a hospice facility.

Because the hospice can accept for care only those patients who are certified as terminally ill, the hospice staff works to help the patient and family come to terms with the death they are facing. In some cases, this may mean assisting the patient and family to see that the patient's affairs are in order. In other cases, it may mean offering counseling and support to help them accept and come to terms with what is happening.

Hospices also provide bereavement service, including listening, counseling, and support groups to the patient's survivors after the death. For more information on hospice programs, see the resources section at the end of this chapter.

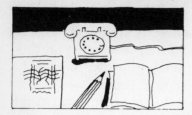

Resources about Working Toward Quality Living

Organizations

Visiting Nurse Associations of America
518 17th Street, Suite 388
Denver, Colorado 80202
303-629-8622

More than five hundred Visiting Nurse Associations exist throughout the United States to provide a variety of home health care services. Check your telephone directory or call the Visiting Nurse Associations of America national office to learn about a Visiting Nurse Association in your locale.

Agencies provide a variety of services, some of which may include hospice and respite programs; homemaker services; speech, physical, and occupational therapy; long-term home health care; nutrition programs/meal programs; and private duty/demand services.

The National League for Nursing
10 Columbus Circle
New York, New York 10019-1350

212-582-1022, extension 248
1-800-847-8480, extension 248
1-800-442-4546, extension 248 (New York State only)

The National League for Nursing operates a toll-free information line to direct individuals to accredited organizations that can provide quality home health care.

National Association for Home Care
519 C Street, N.E.
Washington, D.C. 20002
202-547-7424

An organization that represents all home health care agencies in the United States for legislative and regulatory issues. The association provides a variety of professional and consumer publications through its Foundation for Hospice and Home Care. Contact the Association for its publications list.

The Quality Care National Resource Center
800-645-3633
800-632-3201 (New York State only)
Weekdays 9 A.M. to 5 P.M., (Eastern Standard Time)

Quality Care, a nationwide provider of home nursing services, operates toll-free telephone lines to provide at no charge information about home care and related services. The National Resource Center can provide resource information on home nursing services, hospices, skilled nursing, and rehabilitation facilities, as well as homemaker services in communities throughout the United States. It uses its network of more than two hundred offices for referral information. The Quality Care National Resource Center telephone lines also can provide some information about the locations of specialty programs for cancer patients.

Foundation for Hospice and Home Care
519 C Street, N.E.
Washington, D.C. 20002
202-547-6586

A nonprofit research and consumer-oriented organization that can provide low cost publications, general consumer advice, and support to help in the search for quality home care.

**National HomeCaring Council Division
of the Foundation for Hospice and Home Care**
(Formerly the National HomeCaring Council)
519 C Street, N.E.
Washington, D.C. 20002
202-547-6586

An organization that serves the homemaker and home health aide field. The organization has two books for sale: *Caring for Cancer Patients—A Handbook for the Homemaker-Home Health Aide*, 1986, $6.95; and *Caring for Cancer Patients—A Training Manual*, 1986, $30.

The National Hospice Organization
1901 North Fort Myer Drive, Suite 307
Arlington, Virginia 22209
703-243-5900

This national organization serves as a clearinghouse for information about the fifteen hundred hospice care programs serving the terminally ill throughout the country. The National Hospice Organization offers services including referrals to hospice care in local communities, publications for families and health professionals, an inquiry line for individuals with questions about services and care, and a reference library about hospice care, death, and dying.

Publications include the monthly National Hospice Organization *Hospice News*, the quarterly *Hospice Journal* and *Hospice Team Quarterly*, and the *Guide to the Nation's Hospices*.

Hospice Association of America
214 Massachusetts Avenue, N.E., Suite 240
Washington, D.C. 20002
202-547-5263

The Hospice Association of America, a membership organization for providers of hospice services, can provide patients and their families referral information for hospice, home care, and long-term care.

The National Coalition for Cancer Survivorship
323 Eighth Street, Southwest
Albuquerque, New Mexico 87102
505-764-9956

A national network of organizations that addresses the specific needs of cancer survivors. (Cancer survivors, as defined by the coalition, include all persons with a history of cancer from the time of cancer diagnosis onward.) The coalition serves as a clearinghouse for information, publications, and programs for organizations; as a voice for the issues of survivorship; as an advocate for the rights of survivors; and as a means of promoting the study of survivorship.

Books

Making Peace With Yourself, Harold H. Bloomfield, M.D., with Leonard Felder, Ph.D., Ballantine, New York. $3.95.

Individuals can be trapped by their pent-up feelings of hurt and anger about their own shortcomings. Whatever the negative thinking may be about—dissatisfaction with the way we look, anger when we make mistakes, hurt when someone disappoints us, resentment when we are criticized, living life in a frenzy or feeling unfulfilled in the present and focused on the future—they can be examined and turned into possibilities for personal growth, change, and development.

The authors provide vivid case studies and practical techniques to take charge of our own happiness and life satisfaction by accepting ourselves as we are and allowing ourselves the freedom to give up some behaviors in exchange for new ways of thinking and acting. The rewards are happier, stronger, and more satisfying relationships with ourselves and other key persons in our life.

Making Peace With Your Parents, Harold H. Bloomfield, M.D., with Leonard Felder, Ph.D., Ballantine, New York. $3.95.

This practical, self-help book gives useful advice for working through the stockpile of resentments, anxieties, and hurts we may have involving our parents to achieve a positive, loving relationship with them. The authors use case studies and offer step-by-step techniques for improvement in such areas as "From Resentment to Forgiveness," "Expressing Anger and

Love," "Martyrs, Dictators and Other 'Difficult' Parents," "Unraveling the Sexual Message," "Dealing with Parental Aging, Dying and Death," and "Becoming Your Own Best Parent."

The authors stress the value of working out these key relationships, whether your parents are actually still alive or not, because of the tremendous impact old hurts and resentments can have on a person's current relationships, health, and well-being.

Mind as Healer, Mind as Slayer: A Holistic Approach to Preventing Stress Disorders, Kenneth R. Pelletier, Delta, 1977.

Mind as Healer, Mind as Slayer is a clear, and somewhat technical book that puts special focus on preventive health care techniques that persons can learn and practice to achieve harmony between mind and body. Pelletier offers detailed information for learning ways to exert control over stress reactions through meditation, biofeedback, visualization, and autogenic learning.

This preventive health information may be vitally important. Pelletier describes how stress is implicated as a threat to the normal functioning of body organs and systems, including the immune system. He presents basic findings about controversial topics including the relationship between stress and disease, and he describes certain lifestyles that, he thinks, seem to dispose individuals to certain diseases, including cardiovascular disease, cancer, rheumatoid arthritis, and migraine headaches.

Many readers can benefit from taking responsiblity for their own health. They can participate in their wellness by learning techniques that elicit feelings of well-being and calmness, in addition to providing some control over certain stress reactions and body responses. Pelletier's message: a holistic health view offers opportunities for personal growth and development, self-understanding, a desire to drop self-destructive ways of living and an appreciation for living in the present moment.

Home Health Care: A Complete Guide for Patients and Their Families,
Jo-Ann Friedman, Norton, 1986. $22.50.

This resource book for patients and families is a comprehensive and informative guide to home health care. It offers practical information for managing post-surgical recovery periods as well as daily events living with a chronic illness.

The book provides information about such topics as how to find home health care services and products, how to organize the home to care for the sick person, what services can be expected from home health care aides or therapists, how to set up a support network, and how to determine what Medicare, Medicaid, and private insurance plans will pay.

The Home Health Care Solution: A Complete Consumer Guide, Janet Zhun Nassif, Harper & Row, 1985. $17.95 cloth, $9.95 paper.

The Home Health Care Solution is a resource book with information and step-by-step guidelines on using home care services. This guide describes what home care is and provides guidance on payment options, ways to save on the cost of services, what hospice programs provide, emergency response systems available for patients, and alternatives to home care.

On Death and Dying, Elisabeth Kübler-Ross, M.D., Collier Books, Macmillan, New York, 1970.

Dr. Ross, a psychiatrist, shares terminally ill patients' own words and feelings about accepting their own death. These stories were collected in taped interviews during seminars for students of religion, philosophy, sociology, medicine, nursing, psychology and other disciplines to learn about the experience of death and dying from those who were closest to it. Dr. Ross examines in detail the emotional stages that persons experience when coping with their own or a loved one's death, and clarifies these stages with examples of the reactions of patients who participated in the interviews.

The case studies depict how patients, their families, and health professionals are affected by the reality of death. The stories describe the isolation and hopelessness, as well as the peace and acceptance, that can come when death is imminent.

The author, with the hospital chaplain, demonstrates how listening to and talking with patients in their final days and weeks can expand communication to aid the patient, the family, and health professionals in acceptance of death without guilt or resentment.

Death: The Final Stage of Growth, Elisabeth Kübler-Ross, M.D., A Spectrum Book, Prentice-Hall, Englewood Cliffs, N.J., 1975.

This book is a collection of essays that explores death and dying from a variety of different authors' perspectives. All of the essays highlight the message that death and dying can be a force for new beginnings, creativity, growth, faith, and understanding rather than just a traumatic, destructive experience of pain, separation, and endings.

The essays present opportunities for further thought about the relationship of hospitals and dying persons, perspectives on death in several different cultures and religions, an exploration of how funerals could be managed to better aid the grieving, views about life and death from dying patients, and other inspirational essays concerning the value that death can have to allow one to appreciate life and to experience it fully.

Booklets

"When Cancer Recurs: Meeting the Challenge Again," U.S. Department of Health and Human Services, National Institutes of Health, NIH Publication No. 85-2709.

A booklet for those facing recurrence of cancer with useful reviews of information about diagnosis, treatment, coping suggestions, and resources for getting help.

"Advanced Cancer: Living Each Day," U.S. Department of Health and Human Services, National Institutes of Health, NIH Publication No. 84-856.

A booklet for patients, families, and friends of those facing terminal illness that discusses ways of coping with loneliness, pain, fear of death, and lack of self-respect. The booklet examines common reactions of others to the situation and offers information about financial and legal problems. References and resources are included.

"A Consumer Guide to Home Health Care," Barbara Coleman, Program Coordinator, National Consumers League, 815 15th Street, N.W., Suite 516, Washington, D.C. 20005, 1985. $4. Telephone: 202-639-8140.

A booklet that describes services available under the term "home health care," the personnel who provide these services, the costs for services, and the standards that govern agencies providing services. The booklet provides case studies, a list of questions that enables you to be a savvy consumer of home health care services, and a list of agencies that can provide additional resources and information.

"How to Select a Home Care Agency," National Association for Home Care, 519 C Street, N.E., Washington, D.C. 20002.

This booklet is a guide for consumers selecting a home care agency. Topics covered include, "What Is Home Care?," "How Do You Find Home Care Services?," "How Is Home Care Paid For?," and "Getting the Most from Home Care." The booklet also provides questions to ask yourself, the home care agency, professional and client references as well as questions home care providers may ask potential patients.

A resource list with addresses and telephone numbers of state home health associations is provided.

"A Consumer Guide to Hospice Care," Barbara Coleman, Program Coordinator, National Consumers League, 815 15th Street, N.W., Suite 516, Washington, D.C. 20005, 1985, $4.

This clear and easy-to-read booklet explains what a hospice is, the kinds of services hospices offer, when a hospice program is appropriate, the different kinds of hospice organizations, standards for evaluating hospice programs, general principles about payment for hospice care, and two case studies of families who used the hospice program services. The booklet also includes a checklist with questions for patients and families to ask themselves and to use when gathering information about a particular hospice program.

"Hospice Benefits Under Medicare" is available from your local Social Security Administration office. Ask for publication HCFA- 02154 to learn more about benefits and guidelines for hospice care for persons having Medicare benefits.

Magazines

Cope Magazine
P.O. Box 54679
Boulder, Colorado 80321-4679
1-800-343-COPE
303-238-5035 (in Colorado)
Hours: 8 A.M. to 5 P.M., (Mountain Standard Time),
Monday-Friday

Cope is a news magazine for cancer patients, their families, and physicians. This publication provides news and analysis about developments in the fight against cancer compiled from international news sources.

Cope is not presently sold on newstands. A yearly subscription is $20; two years, $35. Volume discounts of 10 percent are available on orders of ten or more subscriptions.

CHAPTER ELEVEN

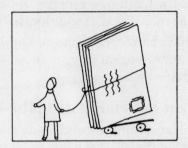

Practical Tips for Handling the Bills

In my practical, no-nonsense moments, I feel that the most useful preparation I had for the experience of fighting cancer was the week I spent a dozen years ago as a temporary employee processing claims for a health insurance company. I learned the basic rules that had to be followed to turn hospital or doctors' bills into reimbursement checks.

Here are guidelines to make the job of handling the bills easier and seeing that you or your doctor gets the check on time. These general guidelines provide tips for dealing with a private insurance company and the Medicare program.

PRIVATE INSURANCE PLANS

Getting the Plan Booklet

As soon as possible after you learn of your illness, request a new, current copy of the plan booklet from your health insurance carrier. Plans change frequently, so do not rely on an old copy in your file.

If you are employed by (or retired from) a company that offers group health insurance coverage, contact the Personnel/Human Resources office or the Employee Benefits Department. Ask your supervisor for assistance if you cannot locate the office.

If you do not have employer-sponsored health insurance coverage, call your insurance agent or insurance provider directly to get the plan booklet.

What to Look for When Reading the Plan Booklet

Read the plan booklet completely and study it carefully. It is the final word on whether the bills get paid, and if so, to what extent. Be sure to find information on the following specific areas:

☐ What is the deductible that must be satisfied before the insurance carrier will begin to reimburse you for medical expenses or pay the doctors or hospitals? This deductible figure is frequently in the $50-200 range, depending on your insurance coverage.

☐ What are the maximum "out-of-pocket expenses" that you will be required to pay after the yearly deductible has been satisfied?

☐ What is the percentage of hospital and non-hospital charges your carrier will pay? These percentages are frequently in the 80 percent to 100 percent range, depending on your coverage.

☐ What, if any, is the percentage of charges for mental health-related expenses that your carrier will pay and what are the yearly or lifetime maximums? These percentages are frequently in the 50 percent range, with $1,000 or $1,500 yearly maximums fairly common, depending on the policy.

☐ What, if any, are the requirements and/or special reimbursement arrangements for obtaining a second doctor's opinion concerning suggested surgery? Many insurance carriers, in their effort to reduce the rising cost of health care, will reimburse fully the cost of getting a second opinion about any proposed surgery.

☐ What is the lifetime maximum the insurance company will reimburse?

Keeping Records Handy

Locate your health insurance identification card provided by the insurance carrier or write down for safekeeping the group or personal health insurance account number if your insurance company does not provide an I.D. card. Begin a folder, file, or portfolio where you keep a full supply of blank health insurance claim forms, your plan booklet, and copies of all your previously submitted claim forms.

At the top of your copy of each claim form you are submitting, jot down for ready reference who the service provider was, the amount to be paid, and the date the claim form was mailed. Be sure to make yourself a copy of everything you submit for payment. Staple your copy of the claim form to your copy of the invoice of charges for easy future reference.

Processing the Claim Forms

Some doctors and hospitals insist on processing the claim forms for you; others will process claims for you as a service if you want it; some leave the entire job to you. Those that automatically handle the paper work for you will require basic information and your signature to start the process. If you do turn over responsiblity for submitting the insurance claim forms to the hospital or doctor's office, check to make sure you will receive copies of all the charges and the claim forms submitted to the insurance company.

Whenever possible, ask the doctor's assistant for the amount of charges for which you can expect to be billed. This will make it significantly easier for you to match insurance payment explanation notifications from your insurance carrier with the statements of charges from the doctor or hospital.

Your insurance carrier will respond to your claim form with a statement that tells what benefits are eligible for payment, have been paid and when, and to whom they were paid. A brief explanation may be provided if no benefits are deemed eligible for payment.

Keeping Track of Your Expenses

Keep every insurance payment statement form, match it to your copy of the claim form and invoice, and staple them together for easy future reference.

Keep a chart with a running total of your out-of pocket expenses. These are the medical expenses that you must pay because part or all of them are not reimbursed by your insurance carrier. Record the service provider and description of the service, the date of service, the amount you are required to pay, and the amount, if any, that the insurance carrier paid.

For example:

Date of Service	Service Provider	Description	Amount Carrier Paid	Amount I Paid

Medical expenses that are not reimbursed by the insurance carrier may be deducted from your income tax if medical bills exceed a certain percentage of your adjusted gross income. If you keep a running total of your out-of pocket medical expenses, it will simplify your work at tax time.

If Your Insurance Claim Is Rejected

If you have difficulty receiving payment for a health insurance claim, do not accept the rejection as final. Make sure that you review your claim form to check that you completed the paperwork correctly. You may want to check that your health provider submitted sufficient information about your case to the insurance company.

If none of this is the reason for denying payment of your claim, begin to contact by phone and in writing the necessary individuals. If your policy is part of a group policy provided by your employer, start with your company's health benefits/human resources office. If you have your own individual policy, contact your insurance agent. After these attempts, contact individuals at the insurance company directly.

While you most likely will need to begin with the claims representative who processed and denied your claim, be prepared to contact the claims supervisor and manager at that office. Eventually, you may need to call or write the corporate office to speak with a claims manager there, as well.

Keep accurate records of all your phone contacts and written correspondence about the rejected claim. If your appeal within the company is unsuccessful and you feel strongly about your case, you can submit a complaint to the state insurance department or take the issue either to small claims court, if small amounts of money are at stake, or to an attorney for large claims.

A number of attorneys will analyze your complaint free of charge. Most accept cases like this on a contigency fee basis. This means that you make an arrangement where the attorney pays all costs and expenses associated with the case and looks to the amount, if any, recovered in the lawsuit to cover the fee. Generally, in a contigency fee arrangement, the lawyer receives one-third of whatever is recovered.

Laws relating to insurance vary from state to state. In some states, patients can sue to recover only the benefits under the policy, while other states allow patients to ask for recovery of damages due to mental and emotional distress.

Refer to the book *Payment Refused* by William M. Shernoff for more detailed information about how to proceed when legitimate health claims are rejected. See the resources section at the end of this chapter for publication information.

MEDICARE INSURANCE PROGRAM

Medicare is a federally-run insurance program that is financed through Social Security taxes. This national program, which is consistent from state to state, provides basic protection against large health care bills. However, Medicare does not pay all health care costs.

How to Know if You Are Eligible

Those who are sixty-five years of age or older, or otherwise eligible for Social Security, are eligible for Medicare benefits. Contact your local Social Security Administration office if you have questions about your eligibility for Social Security or Medicare benefits. Check the telephone number in your local directory. You may find additional useful information in *Your Medicare Handbook,* publication HCFA-10050, which you can request from the Social Security Administration office.

Parts A and B of Medicare Coverage

Medicare coverage is divided into two parts—Part A, Hospital Insurance, and Part B, Medical Insurance. Everyone who is eligible for Social Security benefits is automatically enrolled for coverage in Medicare's Part A, Hospital Insurance. Coverage for Part B, Medical Insurance, for doctors' services, outpatient hospital services, home health care, and other medical services and supplies, is voluntary and, like private health insurance coverage, requires the payment of a premium.

Medicare payment rules and premium costs change frequently, so be sure to check with your Social Security Administration office for current information. Here are some basic facts about the program.

Payments for Medicare Part A, Hospital Insurance, are handled on a set fee arrangement from Medicare directly to the participating hospital. Payments are based on the patient's "diagnosis related grouping." (also referred to as "DRGs") Every patient's illness is categorized into one of more than four hundred and fifty diagnosis related groupings. (There is an "Other" category and exceptions and appeals can be made.) Payments for Medicare Part A are processed by organizations under contract to the government, called "intermediaries," who reimburse the hospital or health care facility a set amount based on the patient's diagnosis.

Medicare Hospital Insurance can help pay for many of the costs of up to ninety days of in-patient hospital care, but insurance deductibles apply for the ninety-day period and even for individual days of hospitalization. Check current Medicare regulations carefully to know the extent of the coverage you can count on.

Medicare Part B, Medical Insurance, is based on a reimbursement to the physician or the patient based on the doctor's reasonable cost. Medicare's Medical Insurance is voluntary, with enrollment requiring a premium payment. (The cost of the premium is set by Congress and is based on a percentage of the program's costs.)

Medicare's Part B requires the fulfillment of a yearly medical insurance deductible. Benefit payments are limited to 80 percent of approved charges.

If you have private health insurance to supplement Medicare coverage (often referred to as "Medigap" coverage), contact your insurance company or agent to find out if your private health insurance policy will cover deductibles, co-insurance costs, or other costs that Medicare does not cover.

Doctors Who Participate with Medicare

Doctors who are "Medicare-participating" have agreed to accept the Medicare payment as payment in full for all approved services. A directory is available that lists Medicare-participating doctors. "Medicare-Non-participating" physicians require that patients make up the difference between the amount the physician charges and the amount Medicare reimburses.

Medicare Coverage and Hospice Care

Individuals who are eligible for Medicare coverage can elect hospice benefits instead of their standard Medicare benefits. In order to select hospice benefits, patients must be certified by their doctor and the hospice medical director as having six months or less to live. The patient also must sign a statement electing hospice care benefits and acknowledging that all of their care must be provided by the hospice program.

If the patient improves and is discharged from the care of the hospice or if the patient needs care outside of the hospice program, the patient can revoke the hospice benefits and go back to the standard Medicare benefit. The patient can do this a total of three times and still have the Hospice Care benefit reinstated at a later point.

The Hospice Care benefit is a lifetime maximum of two hundred and ten days. These days are divided into three benefit periods (ninety days; ninety days; thirty days). Patients forfeit the balance of days remaining in their benefit period when they revoke their Hospice Care benefits in favor of the standard Medicare benefits.

Hospice Care benefits as part of Medicare were new as of mid-1986. Contact your local Social Security Administration office for current information and printed materials. See the resources section at the end of this chapter.

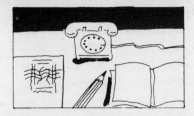

Resources for Handling the Bills

Contact your health insurance carrier for an up-to-date copy of your health insurance plan booklet. Ask your insurance agent or company personnel/human resources office for assistance in getting the plan booklet.

If you are having trouble finding money to pay for the bills, contact your local Cancer Information Service, which may be able to direct you to community agencies that could provide assistance. Use their toll-free line—1-800-4-CANCER. Many nonprofit organizations such as the local offices of the American Cancer Society, The Leukemia Society of America, or the United Cancer Council will also try to assist the cancer patient or family in locating available resources from public and private agencies at the national, state, or local levels.

Many of these nonprofit organizations may also have a staff member or volunteer who can help you file health insurance claim forms if you need assistance and have no one else who can help.

Contact your local Social Security Administration office for information about your eligibility for Medicare benefits or Hospice Care benefits. Check your local telephone directory for the number of the field office serving your area.

Books

Payment Refused, William M. Shernoff, Richardson & Steirman, $16.95. William Shernoff, an attorney who specializes in handling insurance cases, gives practical advice for getting legitimate claims paid even when they have been rejected for payment by the insurance carrier.

The insurance experts at his California-based law firm of Shernoff & Levine analyze a problem free of charge. Many times they find they can give free advice over the telephone to help solve the problem. Contact the firm for more information at 714-621-4935.

Booklets

"Your Medicare Handbook," publication HCFA-10050. Request this booklet from your local Social Security Administration office to learn more about the specific benefits and requirements of Medicare.

"Hospice Benefits Under Medicare," publication HCFA-02154. Request this booklet from your local Social Security Administration office to learn more about the specific benefits and guidelines associated with Hospice Care benefits.

CHAPTER TWELVE

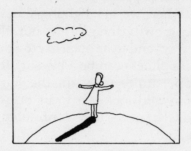

Lessons Learned from the Experience

As I look back on my recent experience of fighting cancer, it is clear to me that I learned a great deal from this frightening and life-threatening ordeal. My life has been enriched and is better and healthier, in many respects, than it ever was.

Priorities change; relationships change; respect for health changes. Life, stripped to its essentials in the fight for survival, provides an atmosphere in which values shift, just as the definitions of accomplishment and success change. The intensified desire to take good care of the body and get well reinforces the drive to grow emotionally and spiritually from the experience.

Many challenges confront the person with cancer or recovering from it. Health issues and the fear of recurrence continue to loom large for a while and only slowly recede.

Another major challenge during the recovery period is to keep a spunky will to live on guard against any and all attackers. This challenge means forging and maintaining new ways of relating, coping, and behaving that support one's will to live. It takes a lot of hard work, but living a full, rich life is worth it.

Using Illness as an Opportunity for Change

Personal growth often happens at a time of hurt, change, or turmoil. The period when we are fighting illness can be one of significant personal growth when we give ourselves permission to look at life in new ways and to be open to growth and change. In a number of instances, illness can be a blessing for those who will seize it as an opportunity to begin the hard work of self-examination. The inward look can focus on what is good and worth keeping and what needs to be confronted, reshaped, or cut loose to be left behind.

I began the lengthy process of closely scrutinizing all aspects of my life three or four months after my cancer diagnosis. *Every* priority, every aspect of my life—professional work, work within the home, social activities, and relationships with family and friends—was examined thoroughly to determine if each was something truly important to me. I decided that "shoulds" need not have ultimate power over my decisions. I opted instead for determining what was really important to me—what I wanted to do, learn, and achieve with my time and energy.

Based on those ground rules, I began the process of making changes. I eliminated responsibilities that sapped my strength and gave few meaningful rewards in return. I changed jobs within the company in order to leave behind me an experience that had proved costly to my health. I decided to stop polishing an already sparkling clean house. I limited my social activities to those I thought would produce enjoyment rather than just keep me involved in a busy social life. I decided to calculate in advance the amount of time and emotional energy I would allot to a particular volunteer activity when I agreed to be involved in it. As I worked on the project, I limited my time to that pre-determined amount.

I added a social service dimension to my life that brought me in contact with caring people and gave me a sense of personal accomplishment and worth. Also, I set aside time each day and evening when I would not be interrupted by family or friends to let my body relax and restore itself through meditation or relaxation response. I decided to push against the limitations of my life by being willing to listen to others around me, including professional therapists, who could assist me to be open to changing and doing things differently.

Adding the Word "No"

For the first time in my life, I took responsibility for using my time as I wanted it to be used. This significant change meant adding the word "no" to my vocabulary and realizing that good friends, family, and even supervisors can come to understand and accept this honesty. This decision meant having to confront, politely but firmly, out-of-towners who were accustomed to having my home as their "home away from home." This change meant eliminating those things from my life that were unhealthy—like overworking and "undersleeping"—and adding those things to my life—like exercise and laughter—that strengthened my body and spirit.

I learned from the experience of cancer that careful self-examination needs to be a constant part of life. Fighting cancer helped me realize the value of this self-scrutiny and gave me permission to examine my life, respond to what I saw, and revolutionize the way I live.

The Value of Expressing Feelings

Another lesson I learned from the experience of fighting cancer is that good health demands that relationships be good, solid, honest ones. Without this, life has a hollow ring to it. Honesty means we need to determine how we feel about important things and then openly express those feelings to the key persons involved in the issue. For the short term, this experience may be unpleasant, but it is a wise investment in long-term health and well-being.

Before my cancer diagnosis, it was common for me to ignore or put aside both small and large issues that made me disgruntled or unhappy. I often decided not to confront another person about the difficulty or shortcoming in our relationship. I preferrred to put aside how I felt in order to keep our relationship going along pleasantly. It seemed simplest to live with problems quietly, not to initiate any conflicts, and keep the day-to-day interchanges unruffled.

I learned the hard way that putting such a gloss on the outside gnaws away at the inside. I learned that all relationships have conflicts and that facing up to these conflicts honestly and working through these disagreements openly is a vital, valuable part of allowing the relationship to be healthy and ever-changing. If we are willing to take some short-term pain and conflict by confronting others honestly, we can enhance the long-term health and vitality of our relationships.

Confronting Rather Than Ignoring a Problem

I learned to develop a workable strategy for ensuring that I examine, rather than ignore, important issues openly and honestly. First, I have learned to acknowledge that a problem exists and decide that I'm going to work toward resolving it. Next, I determine what that problem is and whom I need to talk with or what I might do to help resolve that problem. Most important at this time is my decision that I will not conceal the problem, but will work with someone else to help find a solution. I brainstorm solutions that I think may work and talk with the person to get his or her ideas and share my own suggestions for ways that the problem might be resolved.

This technique is basic good sense. It is difficult to follow at first, because it requires confronting another individual about difficulties. Even though it is easier in the short run to quietly tolerate an unpleasant experience in order to keep the peace, this approach is hazardous to health and happiness.

I recently had a problem to which I applied this step-by-step approach when my work responsiblities required many late nights and much weekend work. After talking with a close friend and a counselor about the demands at work, I was able to see that my response of overworking was really an example of my attempt to ignore the problem in the workplace by keeping myself busy with a frantic work pace.

Once I gained this insight, I decided to develop a solution to confront the problem honestly rather than live with it. I analyzed the problem and determined that I needed more equipment, staff, and support from my supervisor to resolve the problem. Then I went to my supervisor to discuss the difficulties and suggest solutions.

For the short term, the experience was unpleasant—telling my supervisor that a problem existed, asking for his cooperation and support, and not getting it. But I went back to him with additional facts to support the same message, and eventually he came to accept my honesty and the need for additional support. Despite the short-term discomfort of confronting the problem, the long-term impact of these changes made for a happier, healthier work environment.

Taking Good Care of Ourselves

Another important lesson I learned from the experience of fighting cancer is that the only way to take good care of ourselves is by taking on that responsiblity. This sounds obvious, but my experience throughout life—at home, at work, at church—had led me to believe that what mattered was taking good care of family or friends and being responsible for keeping others happy.

I learned through the illness that our first responsiblity is to look within ourselves to realize that we are worth the effort to make ourselves happy and then to see that we do take care of ourselves and allow ourselves to find that happiness. Only when we have allowed ourselves to look within to find and develop peace and happiness do we have something we can share with others that they will enjoy, too.

Because of the experience of fighting cancer, I learned that I am responsible first and foremost for taking care of myself, and that I need to become the expert on this particular subject. Now when family and friends suggest that they know what is best for me and what will make me happy, I greet their suggestions skeptically. I have learned that I have to take care of my body and mind and refill its energy supply each day in a variety of ways, such as through exercise, relaxation response, recreational activities, meditation, or quiet time.

I learned that my constant, harried activity and my desire and ability to pack twice as much as possible into each day to help and serve others at work and at home was a costly lifestyle that did not foster taking care of myself, and eventually became a threat to my health.

I learned how to make non-negotiable decisions to take care of myself. I started my personal, emotional reserve savings bank where I could accumulate those healthful things that give pleasure and renew and restore my body and mind. I insure the accumulated wealth in the emotional savings bank by taking an active role in determining my activities and allowing time each day for my body and mind to be refreshed.

Essentially, I have learned that only I know best about what is good for me and what makes me happy. I cannot know this by listening to or following someone else's ideas or by just taking on responsibilities for others' well-being. The only sure way to take care of myself is by heeding those messages that come from deep within.

Being Scared Is Okay

Going through the experience of fighting cancer and recovering from it is hard work, but it's worth it. But besides being hard work, fighting cancer is a scary experience. The popular but inaccurate attitude is that getting cancer means you're going to die. Despite rising survival rates, that pervasive attitude, in itself, makes the experience frightening and almost paralyzing.

For example, the popular press insists on calling us "victims" rather than "patients," "survivors," or "individuals who have cancer." And yet, patients and doctors know that those who put their energy into getting well can make use of the tremendous resources that exist for recovering and for leading a high-quality life after the cancer diagnosis.

Still, the experience with cancer means that each of us at various times throughout the journey will experience those normal, human reactions of being scared of the disease, of the treatment, or of facing an uncertain future in ailing health. It's normal to have moments when you come face-to-face with these fears.

I confront these fears and uncertainties on the anniversaries of my cancer surgeries, on my three-month check-ups with the surgeon and medical oncologist, and on those occasions when I hear news of friends, acquaintances, or celebrities who have succumbed to cancer. These periodic and passing fears are normal and are to be expected.

Life After Cancer

The struggle one faces in order to live a high-quality life while recovering from cancer is to find that ideal balance between the extremes of denying the past illness and over-concentrating on the current or future state of health. It's vital to be alert and aware of the increased risks of the recurrence of cancer, yet it's also essential

LESSONS LEARNED FROM THE EXPERIENCE

to live fully and without a constant dread of recurrence looming over you.

One way to try to achieve this ideal balance of easy acceptance of one's current state of health is to see that doctor visits or check-ups are on schedule and that any messages the body sends out are considered, watched, and reported to the doctor, if necessary.

Besides this, the essential element is to live joyfully and hopefully, to enjoy the present moment and look ahead to a bright future.

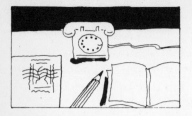

Resources for Lessons Learned from the Experience

Books

One Minute for Myself, Spencer Johnson, William Morrow, 1985.

One Minute for Myself, a parable about a young person's search for happiness in personal and business relationships, teaches simple but often overlooked truths. The basic message of the book is that taking better care of and being nicer to yourself results in a positive, less resentful attitude that allows you to love yourself and others.

The simply-written tale illustrates how these basic truths can be incorporated into daily life to make tremendous changes in how people see themselves, relate to others, and have others relate to them.

Women Who Love Too Much, Robin Norwood, Tarcher, 1985.

Women Who Love Too Much describes why people can find themselves repeatedly drawn into painful, disastrous, even addictive relationships. Ms. Norwood uses stories of a number of individuals—men and women—to show that these chaotic, unfortunate situations are not coincidences, but unconscious choices to re-enact and overcome the old, familiar situations and relationships from childhood. The author offers suggestions and real life examples for breaking the addiction to this kind of relationship. While Ms. Norwood is specifically concerned with dysfunctional relationships between individuals, she indicates that many who have an unhealthy pattern of relating are also drawn to professions where they can exercise their "need to be needed" and to help and control others.

How to Survive the Loss of a Love, Melba Colgrove, Ph.D., Harold H. Bloomfield, M.D., and Peter McWilliams, Bantam, 1977.

How to Survive the Loss of a Love offers practical suggestions as well as poetic insights for recognizing a loss and them marshalling forces to survive, heal, and grow from the experience.

A useful lesson for those facing serious illness or its possible recurrence is that illness is a loss—a loss of health—to be recognized and recovered from like other, more obvious losses.

Necessary Losses, Judith Viorst, Simon and Schuster, 1986.

Necessary Losses weaves together insights from literature, poetry, theology, psychiatry, and other disciplines to describe how our lives are shaped by the losses we experience. These losses, and the way we respond to them, provide us the opportunity for growth, gain, adaptation, and fulfillment.

I hope you find that the practical tips, resources, and reminders presented in this book help you achieve that high quality of life that can make fighting cancer a successful and rewarding experience.

These are definitions for technical terms used in this book. Definitions are those commonly used by The National Cancer Institute and/or the American Cancer Society. (Words set in SMALL CAPITALS are defined elsewhere in the Glossary.)

ADJUVANT THERAPY. Treatment used in addition to the primary therapy. Adjuvant CHEMOTHERAPY or adjuvant RADIATION THERAPY would be used in addition to surgery.

BENIGN TUMOR. A growth that is not cancer and does not spread throughout the body.

BIOPSY. Removing tissue surgically to examine it through a microscope in order to determine whether the TUMOR it came from is benign or malignant.

CANCER. A general term for more than one hundred different diseases. Abnormal cells grow uncontrollably and invade and destroy healthy tissues.

CHEMOTHERAPY. A treatment for cancer using anticancer drugs.

HODKGIN'S DISEASE. A form of cancer affecting the lymphatic system.

IMMUNOLOGY. The branch of science dealing with the body's resistance to disease or invasion from a foreign substance.

LEUKEMIA. Cancer of the blood-forming tissues (bone marrow, LYMPH NODES, spleen) characterized by over production of white blood cells.

LYMPH. A clear fluid that circulates throughout the body, containing white blood cells (lymphocytes), antibodies, and nourishing substances.

LYMPH GLANDS or **NODES.** The part of the lymphatic system that produces LYMPH and lymphocytes, which act as filters to remove wastes and carry fluids to fight infection.

LYMPHOMA. Malignant growths of LYMPH NODES.

MALIGNANT TUMOR. A TUMOR made up of cancer cells.

MELANOMA. A highly malignant form of skin cancer.

METASTASIS. The spread of disease from one part of the body to another. Also, metastasis is the term for a secondary CANCER growing at the distant part of the body.

ONCOLOGIST. A physician who specializes in the treatment of CANCER. Oncologists can be surgical, medical, or radiation oncologists.

PDQ—PHYSICIAN DATA QUERY. A computerized database that provides doctors and patients with the latest CANCER treatment information.

PALLIATIVE CARE. Care that eases the pain rather than curing the disease.

PATHOLOGY. The science of the nature, cause, and development of disease through examining body tissues and fluids.

PATHOLOGIST. A physician who is trained to examine cells and tissues for changes.

PROSTHESIS. An artificial replacement for a missing body part, such as a breast, arm, or leg.

PROTOCOL. Standarized procedures for treatment.

RADIATION ONCOLOGIST. A physician specializing in treating CANCER with RADIATION THERAPY.

RADIATION THERAPY. A way of treating CANCER with high-energy rays.

RECURRENCE. Reappearance of CANCER at the same site (local), near the initial site (regional), or in other parts of the body (metastatic).

REMISSION. Complete or partial disappearance of the disease or the period when the disease is under control.

SIDE EFFECT. A secondary and usually unpleasant effect from a drug or other treatment.

TUMOR. An abnormal mass of tissue that serves no useful body function. Tumors are benign or malignant.

X RAY. Radiation that in low levels can diagnose disease and at high-energy forms can treat CANCER.

Diagnosis, 19, 23, 41
Diagnosis aftershock, 20
Disagreement on diagnosis, 45-46
Discrimination, employment. *See* Employment discrimination
District of Columbia, 50

E

"Eating Hints," 89, 96
Emotional support, 29, 30, 31, 32, 35, 36, 37, 39, 40, 73, 99-113, 117, 123-128, 132-133
Employment discrimination, 24-25
ENCORE, 33, 107
Equipment loan, 28
Europe, 31
Exercise, 33, 130

F

False cheerfulness from others, 125-126
Fear of recurrence, 105, 153, 158-159
"Fight for Your Life," 40
Fighting Cancer, 39
Financial assistance, 22, 30-31, 32, 35-36, 139, 151
Fiore, Neil A., 72, 110-111, 128
Florida, 28, 50, 109
Foundation for Hospice and Home Care, 135
Friedman, Jo-Ann, 139
Funt, Allen, 119, 121

G

Georgia, 28
Germany, 31
Getting Well Again, 37
Goodman, Joel, 119-120, 121
Guestroom Program, 29-30

H

Hair loss, 83, 94
Healing Family: The Simonton Approach for Families Facing Illness, 127
Home health care, 33, 35, 131-136, 141

Home Health Care: A Complete Guide for Patients and Their Families, 139
Home Health Care Solution, The, 139
Home test kits, 21
Hospice Association of America, 136
Hospice care and programs, 132-133, 135-136, 139, 141-142
   Medicare and hospice care, 142, 149-150, 151, 152
Hot Lines, 108-110
"How to Select A Home Care Agency," 141
How to Survive the Loss of a Love, 161
Humor, 115-122
Humor journal, 117
Humor Project, The, 120
Humor workshops, 119-120

I

I Can Cope, 28
Ice cap, 83
Illinois, 50, 51, 58, 59
Imagery, 89, 97
Immunotherapy, 38
Insurance
   claim form processing, 145-146
   I.D. card, 145
   Medicare, 147-150, 152
   plan booklet, 143-144
   Private insurance plans, 143-147
   recording expenses, 145-146
   rejected claims, 146-147, 151-152
Iowa, 59

J

Job discrimination. See Employment discrimination
Johnson, Spencer, 160
Jordan, Hamilton, 42
Journal
   humor, 117
   medical, 20
   emotional, 117

K

Kentucky, 51
Kübler-Ross, Elizabeth, 139, 140

L

Leukemia Society of America, 22, 30-31, 108, 151

Laryngectomy Patient Rehabilitation Program, 29, 107

Laughing Matters, 121-122

Laughter therapy, 115-122

Laughter Therapy, 119

Listening to diagnosis, 19-20

Lost Chord, The, 29, 107

M

Make Today Count, 22, 31, 104, 108

Making changes, 100-102, 137, 153-155, 160

Making Peace with Your Parents, 137-138

Making Peace with Yourself, 137

Maryland, 51, 59

Massachusetts, 51

Mastectomy, 33, 36, 105

McWilliams, Peter, 161

Meals on Wheels, 33, 85, 93-94

Meal service programs, 33, 85, 93-94

Medicare insurance, 147-150
  Social Security Administration, 148, 150, 151-152

Medicare and hospice care, 149-150, 152

Meditation, 130, 138

Michigan, 52, 60

Minnesota, 52

Mind as Healer, Mind as Slayer, 138

Miracles, 105

Missouri, 60, 109

Morra, Marion, 38

Mortality, 131

My Father, My Son, 41, 111

N

Nassif, Janet Zhun, 139

National Association for Home Care, 135

National Association of Meal Programs, 33, 85, 93

National Cancer Institute, 21, 27, 35, 39, 43

National Cancer Institute-designated Cancer Centers, 22, 43, 44, 47-56, 71
  Baltimore, Maryland, 51
  Belmont, California, 49
  Birmingham, Alabama, 48
  Boston, Massachusetts, 51
  Bronx, New York, 53
  Buffalo, New York, 53
  Burlington, Vermont, 56
  Chapel Hill, North Carolina, 54
  Chicago, Illinois, 50, 51
  Columbus, Ohio, 54
  Detroit, Michigan, 52
  Duarte, California, 49
  Durham, North Carolina, 53
  Galveston, Texas, 55
  Hanover, New Hampshire, 52
  Houston, Texas, 55
  Lexington, Kentucky, 51
  Los Angeles, California, 49
  Madison, Wisconsin, 56
  Memphis, Tennessee, 55
  Miami, Florida, 50
  New Haven, Connecticut, 50
  New York, New York, 52, 53
  Philadelphia, Pennsylvania, 54
  Providence, Rhode Island, 55
  Richmond, Virginia, 56
  Rochester, Minnesota, 52
  Rochester, New York, 53
  Salt Lake City, 55
  San Diego, California, 49
  Seattle, Washington, 56
  Tucson, Arizona, 48
  Washington, D.C., 50
  Winston-Salem, North Carolina, 54

National Coalition for Cancer Survivorship, The, 137

National Consumers League, 141

National Council of Jewish Women, 36

National HomeCaring Council Division, 136

National Hospice Organization, 136

National Institutes of Health, 44, 47, 113, 140

National League for Nursing, 134

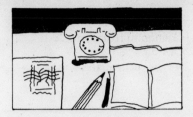

Let Us Know
About Other Resources

If you are aware of other resources that would be useful to patients fighting cancer, let us know. Your resource suggestions will be considered for revising and improving the next edition of this book.

Please print:

Resource name_____

_____

Address_____

_____

_____ ZIP_____

Telephone_(___)_____

Brief description:_____

_____

Optional information:

Your name_____

Your address_____

_____

_____ ZIP_____

Your Telephone_(___)_____

Please return this information to:

Surviving Cancer Resources
P.O. Box 33581, Farragut Station, Washington, D.C. 20033